Identity and Sexuality

AIDS in Britain in the 1990s

Philip Gatter

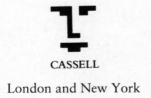

CASSELL

London and New York

Cassell
Wellington House, 125 Strand, London WC2R 0BB
370 Lexington Avenue, New York, NY 10017–6550

First published 1999

British Library Cataloging-in-Publication Data
A catalogue record for this book is available from the British Library.

ISBN 0–304–33341–7

Library of Congress Cataloging-in-Publication Data
Gatter, Philip.
  Identity and sexuality : AIDS in Britain in the 1990s / Philip Gatter.
      p.   cm.
  Includes bibliographical references and index.
  ISBN 0–304–33341–7
  1. Sex role—England—London. 2. Gender identity—England—
London. 3. Gays—England—London—Identity. 4. AIDS
(Disease)—Patients—England—London. 5. HIV infections—Patients—
England—London. 6. Community life—England—London. 7. London
(England)—Social conditions. 8. London (England)—Politics and
government.
  I. Title.
HQ1075.5.G7G37 1999
305.3'09421–dc21   98–30982
                                                              CIP

Typeset by York House Typographic Ltd, London
Printed and bound in Great Britain by The Cromwell Press, Ltd,
Trowbridge, Wiltshire

Contents

Acknowledgements

Writing this book has depended on the support of many during its long genesis. Special thanks go to Rayah Feldman, Pat Warren and Andrew Bebbington, with whom I worked on the research which initially inspired the narrative, and which was funded by the Department of Health. Andrea Cornwall is responsible for suggesting I write a book in the first place. Throughout the frustrations of writing I have been encouraged by Julia Hall, Angie Hart, Cassandra Lorius, Brian Heaphy, Kevin Eisenstadt, Miriam David and Jeffrey Weeks (and my apologies to anyone I've forgotten).

Special thanks are due to Katie Deverell, who took the time to read the draft manuscript of the book and offered many helpful comments for improvement.

Lastly, and most importantly, I must thank all those people who were prepared to share with me their experiences of living with HIV/AIDS, and the Landmark. Without them this book would not have materialized.

Preface

It has long seemed to me unfortunate – and I'm taking the global view here – that such an important experiment in social organization [communism] was left to the Russians when the British would have managed it so much better. All those things that are necessary to the successful implementation of a rigorous socialist system are, after all, second nature to the British. For a start, they like going without. They are great at pulling together, particularly in the face of adversity, for a perceived common good. They will patiently queue for indefinite periods and accept with rare fortitude the imposition of rationing, bland diets and sudden inconvenient shortages of staple goods, as anyone who has ever looked for bread at a supermarket on Saturday afternoon will know. They are comfortable with faceless bureaucracies and, as Mrs Thatcher proved, tolerant of dictatorships. They will wait uncomplainingly for years for an operation or the delivery of a household appliance. They have a natural gift for making excellent jokes about authority without seriously challenging it, and they derive universal satisfaction from the sight of the rich and powerful brought low. Most of those above the age of twenty-five already dress like East Germans. The conditions, in a word, are right.

Bill Bryson, *Notes from a Small Island*

A word concerning what this book is *not*. The subtitle is *AIDS in Britain in the 1990s*. I am an anthropologist (amongst other identities), but this is not really an ethnography in any conventional sense. Though my analysis, both of AIDS and identities, is located in Britain, I am not attempting to define what is culturally specific about the British experience. To do so would require careful cultural interpretation and comparison, a task beyond what I could accomplish with my limited data.

This is an apology, implying a sense of guilt. At conferences it is clear that there is an implicit, and sometimes overt, dominion of Western academic thought about what are the important issues concerning sexuality and AIDS. Most of the references in this book, indeed, are from Western scholars in sociology, cultural studies, politics and lesbian and gay studies. Anthropologists are losing their traditional (professional) reticence over matters sexual, but derive their inspiration (in the main) from cultural worlds far removed from the previously mentioned writers. Rarely do the twain meet. Beyond Boundaries: Sexuality across Culture, a multidisciplinary conference held in Amsterdam in 1997, was a rare exception to this academic tribal separation. The conference fostered interest in debates over such things as the globalization of identities (particularly sexual identities) and the political implications of such globalization alongside economic penetration by the West.

This is all to the good, but a notable gap remains. As Ken Plummer says, reviewing the state of the sociology of same-sex relations, ethnographies of sexualities by Westerners concerning their own societies and cultures remain scarce.[1] My book is an incomplete attempt at such a 'proper' ethnography, and herein lies one of its limitations.

Bill Bryson's cultural stereotype of the British, apart from being hilarious, contains, as all stereotypes do, some truth. But if I can be allowed one unexamined stereotype in response, it is to say that the reaction to AIDS in Britain has been strikingly un-British, with the qualified exception of the sense of pulling together in adversity. Pushed beyond the limits of understatement, we have in our various constituencies been very vocal about what AIDS means in social, cultural, political, identity and medical terms. If nothing else, I hope to have heard and represented some of these voices in what follows.

Philip Gatter
June 1998

Note

1. Afterword to *Social Perspectives in Lesbian and Gay Studies: A Reader* (London: Routledge, 1998).

Introduction

This book is about identities, in particular sexual identities. It explores these identities in the setting of London in the last decade of the twentieth century. It is a contribution to analysing relations between self and community at a time when identity politics, and themes of lifestyle and citizenship, are prominent in reflections on the nature and direction of society in Western countries. It will be of particular interest to students of the social sciences and cultural studies.

The subsidiary theme of the book is AIDS. This is determined not only by the time at which the book is written (AIDS has, unfortunately, been unavoidable in contemporary social analysis); or because the research on which it draws concerns experiences of living with HIV/AIDS and AIDS organizations. As importantly, it is because AIDS can be seen from a social analyst's perspective as a phenomenon that has focused and crystallized many of the dominant concerns about life in contemporary, late modern (or postmodern) society and culture. I hope that what follows will provide a novel insight into some of our current predicaments by explicating identities through an argument about AIDS as a social phenomenon.

Orientations: identities and AIDS

We are at an historical juncture where the end of AIDS is, in some quarters, being confidently predicted. The emergence of new treatments for AIDS-defining illnesses points to a future in which AIDS may become a manageable chronic syndrome, much like other chronic illnesses. This book centres on the experiences of people living with HIV and AIDS in London in the early 1990s, a period in which there was a massive expansion of services for HIV prevention and care, in the context of AIDS being seen publicly as a dread symbol of death. Much of the reaction by and on behalf of those affected by HIV and AIDS at this time can be seen as a response to the equation AIDS = death, which associated a new and potentially terrifying illness with people seen as deviant 'others': gay men, injecting drugs users, black Africans and prostitutes. Stigma, and a demand for resources to combat HIV generally and develop treatments for those directly affected, led to a remarkable series of community mobilizations around HIV/AIDS. The early responses of gay men in Britain, North America and Australia are particularly well documented (see Altman, 1986; Berridge, 1996; King, 1993; Patton, 1990). In New York Gay Men's Health Crisis was established in 1982, campaigning for resources and offering support through buddying. In Britain the Terrence Higgins Trust (THT) was founded, also in 1982, following the death of Terry Higgins, one of the first people to die from AIDS in Britain. It has since become the country's leading voluntary sector HIV/AIDS organization, serving all groups affected by HIV, but with a strong input from gay men.

What began as community-based mobilization became a well-established voluntary sector response to AIDS (Berridge, 1996; King, 1993). Campaigning led the government to accept that the most effective strategy for combating HIV and AIDS was to target resources at the groups most affected, in the context of policy shifts towards care in the community in the late 1980s. In practice this meant that some specialist services at the border between health and social care were to be provided by dedicated voluntary organizations rather than the state, in a quasi-market health care system in which the purchasing and providing of services were to be separated. Statutory health funds were available to voluntary sector organizations who could bid successfully, and competitively, for them. In the HIV/AIDS sector large, generic organizations such as the THT were followed by many smaller groups serving particular constituencies: women, injecting drugs users and ethnic minorities. At the time of our research the voluntary sector organizations operating in London included Body Positive, Positively Women, Blackliners, the

Black HIV/AIDS Network (BHAN) and Mainliners (injecting drugs use).

All these organizations had both advocacy and service provision functions, whether directly or as networks of referral. They existed at the interface between the state, as represented by health and social services, and the person living with HIV/AIDS. In one sense their role was political since they sought to represent the interests of certain groups. But who constituted these groups was not obviously related to traditional political affiliations of party or class. Rather, their memberships were determined by the epidemiology of HIV, a process that linked people through behaviours carrying a risk of the transmission of body fluids and thus not necessarily related to previously existing social, cultural or political links.

This book explores how people have identified themselves in response to the AIDS crisis. Later chapters consider in detail processes of identification; here I wish to signal the diversity of groups affected by AIDS in terms of forms of social linkage. To be a gay man in a city such as London is to be self-consciously aware of belonging to the group numerically most affected by HIV and AIDS. The terms gay community or lesbian and gay community are common currency now, even beyond those who regard themselves as members: when a crime occurs at some site used by gay men cruising, the police are now heard to call on support from the 'gay community' rather than 'homosexuals'. Yet gay community is, to use Jeffrey Weeks's term, a 'necessary fiction'. It is a powerful signifier for identification and solidarity which tends to overwrite diversity. Empirical social research (e.g. Kippax *et al.*, 1993; Vincke *et al.*, 1993) reveals a wealth of forms of attachment to gay community which suggests that 'community' can be used rather as Humpty Dumpty used words, to mean what he chose them to mean. Community has become a weasel word.

'When *I* use a word,' Humpty Dumpty said in a rather scornful tone, 'it means just what I choose it to mean – neither more nor less.'

'The question is,' said Alice, 'whether you *can* make words mean different things.'

'The question is,' said Humpty Dumpty, 'which is to be master – that's all.' (Lewis Carroll, *Through The Looking Glass* [1888], p. 114)

Humpty Dumpty means whether he or the words are master. What I am more interested in is who gets to define the use of terms, how and why. We need to examine how 'community' develops as an analytical term, but in relation to how it is used by people claiming to belong to communities, a subject that is explored in Chapter 4.

London sustains all aspects of a gay life, providing parks and heaths, pubs and clubs, bookshops, a film festival, and the headquarters of a number of campaigning groups, such as Stonewall. In this environment many gay men (and lesbians) have a very well-developed sense of participating in a gay community. The social networks of some London gay men consist largely of other gay men, driven by a sense of needing to belong with others sharing a stigmatized sexuality. These networks exist through the commercial gay scene, gay political and social groups (Lesbian and Gay Switchboard, coming-out groups, gay choirs and orchestras to name a few, as well as HIV/AIDS organizations) and developing friendship networks. Significantly, this version of being gay is powerfully evoked by leading, if self-appointed, representatives of gay community in the arts, media and health. But this is only part of the story. For other gay men, sexuality is more compartmentalized from sense of self, and social and cultural networks are not primarily defined by shared sexuality (Annetts, Eisenstadt and Gatter, 1996; Davies, 1992). And there are further subtleties, such as the queer politics movement, which seeks identification around difference that is not just about a binary hetero/homosexual division. To describe being gay as implying a shared, easily recognizable identity expressed through community is therefore simplistic. In analysing the experiences of young gay Irish men in Britain, Mac an Ghaill finds the complexities theoretically and methodologically challenging:

> As a white ethnic minority, young Irish men occupy a unique social location in which to explore the complexities, ambivalences and contradictions of contemporary forms of sexuality. On the one hand, they are ascribed masculine privileges as White men. On the other hand, as a subordinated masculinity, they experience a constant surveillance in public arenas, with their accent as a key signifier of social identification and cultural difference. (Mac an Ghaill, 1996, p. 122)

To be a member of an ethnic minority has more obvious cultural and social connotations. Religion, a minority language and specific cultural values such as rules regarding marriage may be held in common. Social networks may be primarily with other members of the same ethnic community, and such communities tend to be clustered, mainly in inner-city areas. Community identification and solidarity will also be driven by the experience of racism and discrimination, on the street and in the workplace.

Being a woman, and consciousness of what this means, centres on other sets of issues, and varies between women. Gender-based differences between men and women's access to economic resources and self-determination form a basis for political identification through a number of feminisms. Health has emerged as a feminist issue, since women may have differential access to health care, and suffer some health problems disproportionately (such as anxiety and depression) as well as having distinctive areas of health need that are biologically gendered. These concerns are reflected in the establishment of women-specific services such as Well Woman clinics. Women have distinctive health needs in relation to HIV/AIDS as well, especially gynaecological complications, as articulated by Robin Gorna in *Vamps, Virgins and Victims* (1996).

To be an injecting drugs user does not imply a strong sense of community or shared identity, beyond participating in networks of drug distribution and use. In the popular imagination the injecting drugs user is someone who places himself outside society and community through behaviours that are antisocial (crimes to obtain money for drugs) and who is not a fully conscious being when high on drugs. This is a stereotypical view containing, as stereotypes do, some truth, but also obscuring the diversity of people who have a drug habit: in 1998 the police in Britain were drawing attention to the widespread use of heroin in the middle-class suburbs.

Of course, each of the groups described is not mutually exclusive. Women may be members of ethnic minorities. Gay men may be injecting drugs users. For any individual there are likely to be a number of overlapping identifications, of variable relative importance through time.

Even on a cursory examination we can see that the different interest groups which have formed around AIDS are not equivalent in terms of the substance of the linkage between group members. One response to this might be to view AIDS mobilization in purely instrumental terms.

The epidemiology of HIV marks a number of non-equivalent groups of individuals as being at special risk of exposure to HIV. In the context of limited resources to tackle HIV, it is rational for individuals identifying themselves as members of risk groups to unite in pursuit of resources. The emergence and activities of the various voluntary sector organizations might be seen as simply the sum total of the pursuit of individual self-interest. Unity forged of necessity. If this is the case, then it may be illusory, or at least misleading, to talk of identity at all.

Contradicting this perspective is a great body of social research and cultural criticism, which argues persuasively that AIDS has been a pro-foundly social phenomenon focusing anxieties about the very nature of society at the end of the twentieth century. Those who have come together to form alliances in the face of AIDS have done so precisely because the force of AIDS has been much more than medical. Morally conservative groups have linked AIDS to kinds of people and lifestyles they disapprove, and are fearful of. Fundamentalist Christian sects in North America see AIDS as a punishment from God for the sin of sex outside heterosexual monogamous marriage: 'AIDS is God's judgment of a society which does not live by his rules' (Jerry Falwell, in Seidman [1996], p. 280). Such values have even come to inform some gay men's self-perception. Larry Kramer began to argue (Kramer, 1990) that AIDS somehow was a reward for a decade of sexual self-indulgence which had harmed mutuality among gay men – a fulfilment of a fatalistic and narcissistic attitude of 'eat, drink and be merry, for tomorrow we die'.

Risking a wild generalization here, I would argue that it is a general human impulse to attach meaning to events beyond our control. At the individual level, if we experience misfortune we want to know 'Why me?' At the level of society, we are tempted to blame epidemics on people who are unlike us, and metaphorize illness as an expression of social as much as bodily ills. We need to attribute agency to the human or superhuman. The anthropological record reveals that many non-Western societies impute the causes of misfortune to the malicious agency of other human beings, often in the form of witchcraft (Evans-Pritchard, 1937; Peek, 1991). Even we moderns are uncomfortable with accepting the scientific rationalist view that we are subject to chance, not fate. For if that is the case, disasters have no meaning and our lives may seem entirely con-tingent.

AIDS is our contemporary plague. It often disfigures the body and, until now, was almost certainly fatal. Society has invested AIDS with social meaning. The mobilization around AIDS which has sought to deny and expunge stigma represents what AIDS means, but in so doing restructures rather than denies the social significance of AIDS. To mobilize against the 'othering' of a moral majority means accepting, if revaluing, 'otherness'. So, for the organizations that have grown up around AIDS, as well as for the wider society, it is as much who you are as the virus you have that counts. AIDS has done something dramatic. It has forced an examination of who we are and what are our priorities, especially those of us who are members of at-risk groups. This self-examination, and the accompanying choices we make about who we need to join forces with, are connected with a medical emergency, but, I will argue, the social crisis generated by the eruption of a virus which medicine has not been able to treat is of equal significance. AIDS is indeed acting as a catalyst to changing the ways in which we identify ourselves, drawing on but going beyond previously established senses of being gay men, black, a woman and so forth. We are still these things, but AIDS modifies what they mean.

Although groups for gay men, women, ethnic minorities, have been discussed as if they were entirely separate, many AIDS service organizations, such as the THT and Body Positive, aim to serve all groups affected by HIV and AIDS without prejudice or distinction. Their ethos, in the face of the stigmatization of AIDS, has been to dissolve boundaries between different kinds of people (which, as we shall see, has not been a simple or easy aim). In doing this they have constructed AIDS as a necessarily unifying phenomenon, and forced both those working for and served by organizations to confront and reconsider their sense of difference from others. Part of the argument of this book will be that AIDS is a social phenomenon that has necessitated a debate about who we are and with whom we have common cause.

I am arguing, therefore, that AIDS is a phenomenon operating at the level of the social. At the same time, AIDS is experienced by the individual as illness. AIDS has induced forms of political identification, but it has done more than this. It is an illness, or rather set of illnesses consisting of acute episodes in a chronic history for the individual. Chronic illnesses are characterized by indeterminacy. Onset may be in the form of vague sets of symptoms occurring over a considerable period, making diagnosis retrospective after other possible causes for the symptoms have been eliminated. Prognoses are often unpredictable. Development of illness typically leads to progressive changes in lifestyle in order to manage debilitation. Treatment for chronic illness may centre on maintenance of quality of life in the absence of cures. In this context, sociologists of health and illness have argued that social analysis is a necessary aspect of the understanding of chronic illness. Since the progression of illness will force changes connected with work and social activities, and physical activity more generally, the chronically ill person is faced with having to re-evaluate his sense of self in terms of the loss of valued activities and a profoundly changed future. And these effects do not only play on the ill individual. They will also change the lives of partners, family and social networks. These sets of events also are more than physical in nature. To be a valued member of society in the industrial West implies being an economically and socially productive individual. Illness, especially long-term, represents an incapacity to fulfil this role. The values attached to being well are such that the chronically ill person is likely to internalize feelings of inadequacy, of having lost part of the self. The nature of these changes to self-identity, and how the chronically ill manage them, have become the subject of a growing literature on the 'experience of illness' within medical sociology. There has been a tendency, though, for the individual experience of illness to be treated as logically prior to, and analytically separable from, group and community response to illness. I am attempting instead to illustrate how the two realms have to be understood as interconnected and mutually reinforcing.

The rest of this book is devoted to tracing the ways in which AIDS is a phenomenon of identification, what this tells us about contemporary identities more generally, and, looking in the opposite direction, how we can use social knowledge of AIDS towards better ways of dealing with it, both medically and politically/socially. It is simultaneously intended as a contribution to the social science of identity, and a social scientific contribution to social policy relating to AIDS.

Chapter 2 outlines the methodological perspective on identity I have adopted which, stated most simply, is to regard identity as process rather than essence, entailing an interactive and iterative approach to research. I situate my approach in the anthropological tradition, but do not attempt an exhaustive review of conceptualizations of identity and associated research methodologies. Instead, I argue for the utility of a specific approach. Chapters 3 and 4 are devoted to applying this perspective to individual and group experience of HIV and AIDS. I look first at how individuals perceive changes to their self-conception as a result of their experiences as HIV-positive people; and then at their wider affiliations as members of AIDS-affected communities. The two chapters are closely interlinked since the division into individual and communal experience is to some extent arbitrary, though the focus is slightly different – the chapter on individual experience is more about self-perceptions linking the body with illness (and relates to the medical sociology literature on experience of illness). Chapter 4 moves the focus to how individuals connect with others, given their circumstances, in and against external constructions of them as AIDS victims. Both chapters draw primarily on the author's empirical research, but in the context of other studies and arguments.

Chapter 5 poses a different kind of question. AIDS as a syndrome can be considered as an example of a chronic illness, though perhaps with special characteristics. I explore here how individual experiences of HIV and AIDS reflect what the literature says about other chronic illnesses, to make an argument about how AIDS is different in terms of its disruption to personal biographies. I also consider how the contextualization of personal in social experiences, as set out in the previous two chapters, may differentiate AIDS from other chronic illnesses. In all these chapters I attempt to trace the similarities and differences in experiences of different kinds of people. In large part I am interested in gay men, and how sexuality figures as a distinctive feature of AIDS identification. This perspective is determined pragmatically by the epidemiology of AIDS in London, so that a high proportion of the respondents in our study were gay men. Though the book may be seen as London-centred, it should be borne in mind that some 65 per cent of all HIV cases to date in the UK (1998) have been in London and cumulatively three-quarters of these cases have resulted from sexual transmission between men. Put differently, this means that up to 49 per cent of all HIV cases in Britain have been among gay and bisexual men in London. It will be for others to explore the experiences of other 'risk groups' such as sub-Saharan Africans in detail. In terms of the book's other major theme, identity, it also makes sense to focus on gay men, given that much recent social analysis has pointed to minority sexual identities as typifying late modern urban identifications.

The final chapter is devoted to exploring how the experience of AIDS in

Britain has changed since the early 1990s. It reviews the implications of my analysis and suggests where qualitative social research might go in future, given some significant changes in AIDS as a social phenomenon.

I am looking at AIDS and identity, but before pursuing this task there is a wider context that needs to be sketched, which will parenthesize the arguments of the book. This is to say that AIDS has come about at a particular historical moment that social theorists characterize, at least in the industrial West, as one in which 'traditional' forms of identification are no longer tenable. We live in an age, they argue, where our senses of self and wider community belongings have to be about working out our own narratives, which is both a creative engagement and a perilous journey. AIDS and its meanings have to be situated in the fabric of what is variously termed late modernity or postmodernity.

Identities and AIDS in a time of insecurity

The progressive secularization of society this century is a familiar background to arguments about social disintegration. For the religious, irreligiosity is mirrored in the statistics on divorce, one-parent families, juvenile crime, drug abuse, and the increasing visibility of alternative (in Christian religious terms, sinful) ways of living. Even those professing no religious belief, or positive atheism, have been profoundly influenced by a Judaeo-Christian ethic which informs our polity, implicitly and explicitly. Whatever causes are invoked, from immanent amorality to the alienating effects of social and economic deprivation, the late twentieth century is widely accepted as an era of profound social change. In a morally conservative view, this flux represents a dangerous erosion of morals and ethics. In a more radical view, it offers hope for a more inclusive and humane society. Either way, we no longer have sets of neatly prescribed values and world views which we can rely on as external guides to living (even accepting that those values have often been implacably opposed to each other in the past), unless, as with religious fundamentalists, we invent new moral codes to impose on ourselves and others. Whatever our political leanings and belief systems, the current age is one of insecurity and uncertainty in the absence of life-prescriptions which the demise of tradition entails. Our lives are about developing personal narratives that resist social entropy.

Social analysts see the current *Zeitgeist* in terms of the broad characteristics of the late modern or postmodern age, in other words one in which the rationalist programme of the Enlightenment and ensuing modernity has been seen to fail. Science questioned religion as a basis for understanding the workings of life from the beginning of the modern era; now science itself is seen not to provide a grand narrative that can make full sense of human existence and put us in control of the future of the planet, albeit there have been major advances in areas such as medicine. We inhabit a largely secular world in which the ground rules associated with traditional forms of social belonging are weakened. One consequence of this is a sense of insecurity about who we are and how we should lead our lives ('we' being intended here as an inclusive and unmarked category, most readily identifiable with the post-industrial West). Linked with this sense of social formlessness (or *anomie* to employ a sociological term) is the idea of risk, simultaneously social, cultural and technical. We often hear that we live in a risk society. We are exposed to industrial risks of contamination, notably from the ubiquitous internal combustion engine; to financial risk in a free market of individualism where old forms of social welfare are being eroded. An increasingly technologized world exposes us also to new hazards in the workplace: from more sedentary lives to sick building syndrome to the physical and psychological effects of stress in highly pressured performance-oriented work cultures. A report on risk by the Royal Society led to a major research programme in Britain funded by the Economic and Research Council (Royal Society, 1992), which recognized the relevance of social scientific perspectives, such as in the work of Ulrich Beck and Mary Douglas (Beck, 1992; Douglas, 1992; Douglas and Wildavsky, 1982).

Risks can ambush us at every turn. Risk management has become an activity of daily life for the individual, as for the polity. For individuals this is most apparent in attempts to minimize risks to the self, to mind and body. We may be assaulted by hazards beyond our control, but we can strive to maintain our physical and mental integrity in the face of them. Most bookshops now have Self-Help sections where we are offered salvation in the form of a healthy mind in a healthy body. Regimens of diet and exercise offer the possibility of a body that will resist disease and stave off the effects of aging, even if it can't quite avoid death yet. Manuals deriving from various forms of psychotherapy, conventional and maverick, offer pathways to emotional stability and happiness without the need for any transcendent belief systems. We can heal our lives, or so the authors would claim. Significantly, we can become addicted to these offers of temporary, if not eternal salvation, precisely because of the crisis in knowledge. If we think of diet alone, the scientific evidence and interpretations of it are constantly changing. Until recently, potatoes and alcohol were evil. Now we should gain our calories from high starch foods, and a moderate intake of red wine is protective for coronary heart disease. Even eggs are being rehabilitated, with the suggestion that they do not have a significant effect on blood cholesterol levels. There is always more to learn and a market for the books and Internet resources that teach us.

Some things we can't heal. There are diseases for which biomedicine and health manuals have no conclusive answers. Alzheimer's disease threatens an irreversible decline, usually later in life. Multiple sclerosis can manifest at any time. But these are conditions thought to be largely under genetic control. They have always been with us, though they are of course distressing for the sufferers and their social circle alike. What haunts life and fantasies in the late modern age are infectious agents for which we have imperfect answers. Chief among these are the retroviruses, including HIV, newly recognized agents such as prions, and previously controlled microbes now running riot or causing unprecedented symptoms, such as the streptococci responsible for toxic shock in the so-called 'flesh-eating disease' necrotizing fasciitis. Notable among this last category are antibiotic-resistant strains of tuberculosis, creating a major health crisis in Russia, where many carriers are going untreated and contributing to the epidemic. Even in Britain, with better funding for treatment and public health measures for containment, ever more cases of this classic Victorian scourge are being reported.

In the popular imagination we are entering a time when previous controls achieved through biomedicine are under threat, a doomsday scenario frequently mined in the immensely popular television series The X Files. Here previously innocuous organisms such as common fungi escape their ecological bounds to become fatal infections. Not only are the microbes fatal: they are carried in each episode by individual humans who become agents of infection synonymous with the disease they carry. The 'innocent' fungus is transposed into a visible, wilful source of harm through identification with a human agent. Sometimes these individuals are criminals; more often they are portrayed as innocent vectors, unaware of what they are doing. They have been invaded by a force beyond their control. The ultimate source of the invader is often extraterrestrial, though we are never sure. In this, the series touches on another facet of late modern society: the will to believe in non-human agency in the absence of religion; to wish for an intelligence in the universe other than our own. Such beliefs are perhaps more powerful in, say, New Mexico than in Britain, but the fascination with accounts of alien visitation is much greater in the West now than ever in the past, together with the wish to believe in aliens as the origin of unexplained phenomena, rather than nature.

Of course, in each episode of *The X Files* the two FBI agents, Mulder and Scully, singlehandedly manage to prevent the extinction of the planet, so we can switch off the television relieved and comforted. This is not the case with some real agents of infection. Among the various agents that have confounded medical science, viruses as a class raise the greatest anxieties. Viral particles inhabit the boundaries between organic life and inorganic matter, having the capacity to invade and reproduce, yet also to remain dormant, almost indefinitely in some cases. Hence the continued anxiety about plague pits in Britain where *Yersinia pestis* might reawaken if disturbed, and the recent fear that Saddam Hussein as international bogeyman might attempt to infect the world lastingly with the deadly virus that causes anthrax. Viruses propagate by taking over the genetic machinery of the cell, making more viral DNA instead of the DNA of the host organism, or, in the case of retroviruses, such as HIV, more viral RNA. Viruses take possession of the body. This possession is most frighteningly realized in the way that HIV operates. In itself it does not lead to death, but it removes the defences of the body against other invaders which, rather as in the narratives of *The X Files*, at other times and in other places are usually harmless. One can argue that HIV is a site focusing contemporary anxieties about lack of proper order in the universe (it disrupts conventional ecologies) and the failure of health regimens to protect the body from risks that surround us. It is also associated with disfiguring illness, marking the imperfectibility and mortality of the body.

HIV fits in with the uncertainty and insecurity of the late modern age. Its recognition in the early 1980s may have been historically arbitrary, but the explosion of signification around it (Treichler, 1988) has to be understood as reflecting, and inflecting, a number of concerns peculiar to our time. I have discussed briefly some meanings of viral illness. As important in contemporary thinking is knowledge of how we acquire viruses, which can be located in the notion of the risk society. We know in the case of HIV that it is unlikely to survive for more than about 20 minutes outside the living human body, and that transmission is therefore almost exclusively through direct contact of body fluids between individuals: via sexual contact, sharing syringes for drug injection, blood transfusion, or vertical transmission between mother and child perinatally or via breast-feeding. We think of these activities in terms of the risks attached to them, and attempt to quantify them. What are the chances that one of our sexual partners is HIV-positive? If positive, what are the chances of transmission, depending on the nature and frequency of contact? In the case of sexual transmission, what difference does the use of condoms make to the levels of risk involved? Given that sexual impulses, or the need to use drugs, may be strong, what do we consider to be risks worth taking? This has become a professional as well as personal matter. Actuaries have advised life insurance companies, based on careful assessment of probabilities, to be wary of insuring gay men, who may represent a bad risk. Some insurance companies have followed this advice, much to the anger of gay activists. Of course, this advice is discriminatory in that it doesn't consider individual behaviours; it treats all gay men as if their risk activities were the same. But on a population level it can be argued to be rational, if not reasonable, if most people with HIV also happen to be gay men.

The science of risk has thus taken up HIV as a legitimate concern. Balancing the actuarial example is the way in which risk calculation has entered into the development of primary HIV prevention campaigns. As knowledge of risk has improved with the trajectory of the epidemic, so HIV prevention has become more refined. Lay thinking about HIV is also permeated with the language of risk. Risk of exposure to HIV is one of the most frightening potentials in a society saturated by risk, even if most of the population, in absolute terms, are at very little risk. But lay concepts of risk are often tied up with notions of blame. No one, except perhaps God, is blamed for an earthquake. Yet the idea of blame is often very clearly attached to HIV, blame which is even codified by some nations. In the public health systems of Cuba and Sweden the individual is seen as responsible for putting the public good at risk, so quarantining of the HIV-positive person is acceptable. In the United States supposed deliberate infection of another person with HIV can be treated as attempted murder, and in Britain deliberate infection is in the process of being criminalized, a matter discussed in detail in Chapter 6.

In concluding this introduction to the historical and social contexts in which HIV/AIDS need to be understood, I want to consider further how contemporary social theory points up why notions of HIV risk are bound up with ideas of blame, particularly in relation to sexuality; and why sexuality, through personal and social development, is writ large as a component of our identities, identities which have to be achieved. This will provide a foundation on which to base an argument about the connectedness of AIDS, identities and sexuality.

The first tenet in characterizing the late modern age is its uncertainty and contingency. We have to seek out and mould our own senses of self. A second tenet is that this process of identity formation is not unconstrained: there are features of Western society that are more salient, more determinant of who we can be than are others. Outstanding among these is sexuality.

In the last of his major works, *The History of Sexuality*, Michel Foucault presented an historical understanding of the emergence of sexuality as a key social and cultural concern in the West. In the first of the four completed volumes of his history (Foucault, 1978) he set out polemically to challenge the repressive hypothesis concerning the nineteenth century: that it was an age of prudery and the repression of sexuality. Instead, he insisted, the apparent repressions of the Victorian era were about an ever more focused concern with sexual matters, coinciding with the birth of sexology as a serious scientific endeavour.

> Not any less was said about it [sex]; on the contrary. But things were said in a different way; it was different people who said them, from different points of view, and in order to achieve different results. (Foucault, 1978, p. 27)

Foucault famously pronounced that the idea of a sexual identity did not become fully formulated in the way that we understand it until this time. A number of sexual practices earlier had been condemned by the church, among them sodomy, but these were defined as aberrant behaviours, not aspects of discrete kinds of human being. From the mid-nineteenth century the homosexual (a term defined and first used in 1869) became a defined kind of person rather than an otherwise unremarkable individual fallen into evil. As importantly, the idea of the homosexual came to be more than a construction of medical, psychiatric and juridical thought. The discourse of the homosexual created, to paraphrase Foucault, the subject of which it spoke. In other words, the idea of *being* a homosexual came to be internalized by those who saw themselves as sharing the identified characteristics of this new species of being. Oscar Wilde, through his trials in 1895, became a notable signifier of 'the homosexual'. Through the early years of the twentieth century, being a homosexual or a lesbian began to be reflected in a consciousness of minority status, and the nascence of an identity politics based on homosexuality. In one vein of aesthetic writing, novelists such as Edward Carpenter argued for the artistically ennobling characteristics of 'the other love' and in so doing were being more open than Oscar Wilde about its sexual element (Carpenter, 1894). More overt political identification around what can be termed non-normative sexualities has proliferated and diversified through this century, through various phases that have foregrounded assimilation (we are just like everyone else, except in one aspect of our lives), difference (we are different but have the right to be treated as everyone else) and, most recently, queer politics and theory (a post-modernist attempt to remove, or at least reappropriate, identity labels). This process, beginning with homosexuality, has become a debate involving other forms of non-conventional sexuality, including bisexuality, transsexuality and areas of sexual practice such as sadomasochism.[1]

Foucault's discussion of homosexuality is only one example (albeit a key instance) in the development of his thesis of the emergence of sexuality as a dominant discourse of late or postmodernity in the West. He considers also the increasing role of the idea of population in governance, the instantiation of heterosexual monogamous marriage as the fundamental unit of society, the role of psychiatry and medicine in circumscribing childhood sexuality and forms of sexual 'deviance' other than homosexuality. Without trying to summarize his complex argument, its general implication is that sexuality has come to be seen as the truth of the self, at the centre of our identities as human beings. We are not necessarily fully aware of this truth, and contemporary techniques for exploring the self, most notably psychoanalysis, act as the key for unlocking our sexually premised selves. Foucault sees an historical continuity between the church confessional and the psychoanalyst's couch in the revelation of self.

Other scholars have modified Foucault's insights to analyse the nature of late modern identities, analyses that combine the tenet of fragmentariness with the tenet of the centrality of sexuality. Thus, in his recent work on values and community identification (*Invented Moralities: values in an age of uncertainty*), Jeffrey Weeks says that

> The fragility and hybridity of modern personal identities forces everyone in highly developed societies to engage in experiments in everyday life: to define themselves, their identities and their needs against a shifting landscape. (Weeks, 1995, p. 32)

And at the same time

> our sense of self, the meanings we attach to our lives, are closely shaped by our sense of our sexuality. Sexuality may be 'historic construct' (Foucault, 1979), but it remains also a key site for the construction of personal meaning and social location. (*ibid.*, p. 38)

An historical process has occurred, which locates identities in relation to sexuality but in ways that are always contested. At the historical moment we inhabit now it is, most notably, HIV/AIDS that provides a cultural site through which anxieties about sexuality and identity are focused. This, it is argued (Patton, 1990; Watney, 1987), is why AIDS has become culturally associated in such a strong way in Europe and North America with gay men, beyond the unhappy accident that a virus took told in a particular, sexually interconnected population. Gay men, throughout the twentieth century, had been seen as breakers of sexual, and therefore moral, norms. Now they were seen by some as visiting divine retribution on themselves, or at least suffering the consequences of reckless, risky behaviour, along with injecting drugs users, prostitutes, and in the United States, inner-city blacks and Hispanics: all groups seen as living deviant lifestyles outside the boundaries of an implicit white middle-class suburban norm. With the exception, perhaps, of the drugs users, all these groups are in some respects stigmatized in sexual terms: gay men for being 'perverts', prostitutes for prostituting their bodies and using sexuality commercially instead of matrimonially, and non-whites variously for being sexually animal and potential, if not actual, rapists (especially of white women). In all these groups there is a strong configuration between general 'deviance', being a feared 'other' associated with AIDS, and an element of sexuality. In contrast, a white middle-class teacher who is infected with HIV is unlikely to be a suspect in the AIDS drama, unless, for example, someone discovers she had a sexual relationship with a black African man when on holiday in Uganda. In the analysis which follows in later chapters I will be fleshing out the AIDS–identity–sexuality association in trying to understand why it is that gay men in Britain in some senses have a quite distinctive experience of the AIDS crisis, both as individuals and as members of a community.

What is important about AIDS is not just that it has provided a focus for thinking about sexuality and identity. It has also changed things, particularly the ways in which people develop their identities in common cause with others. Social theorists see AIDS as one particular crisis moment through which the instability of contemporary life is refracted. When faced with crises, we seek points of anchorage with others to stabilize our position in the world:

> Crisis moments force their participants to see a coherence in their sense of the world which ordinary circumstances would not have produced . . . The AIDS crisis dramatized for many of those caught in its wake the pretence of contemporary citizenship, a citizenship that excluded huge numbers of people living with, or confronting the threat of, a ghastly and life-threatening syndrome of diseases. (Weeks, 1995, p. 112)

At a collective level, various alliances have formed around AIDS that relate to contemporary identities. Among these are the service provision organizations mentioned earlier. Those that articulate a political response to denied or partial citizenship include the militant identity politics organizations, such as OutRage! in Britain and Queer Nation in the USA. Such organizations play a part in social organization in response to AIDS, the theme of Chapter 4. But they also play a role in what has been identified as a broader contemporary social process. They are an example of what Foucault has termed a critical community (cited in Rajchman, 1991). These are new formulations of community that come into being through the challenging of the meaningfulness of existing communities. Critical communities open the possibility of new kinds of subjectivity.

Groups such as Queer Nation and OutRage! are candidates for critical communities. They reject the terms on which a person is considered a valid, and valuable, member of society. But they do more than this. In the case, particularly, of Queer Nation, they also reject the terms 'gay' and 'lesbian' and the notion of gay and lesbian communities. They disrupt the signifiers that have most clearly identified non-normative sexualities through the twentieth century. In other words, they attempt to transgress a by now widely accepted dichotomy of sexual identification. Of course, they do not have a monopoly in the debates: others continue to assert the meaningfulness of a lesbian or gay male identity. In North America such identities in the 1970s and 1980s were even inhabited as and argued to be a form of ethnicity, an idea still maintained by some. The point is that these kinds of arguments are examples of the wider contemporary paradox of identities being needed to maintain a sense of self, whilst being constantly under scrutiny and subject to reformulation. Jeffrey Weeks has argued that contemporary identities are marked as being heterogeneous, with the possibility of identification across many previously impermeable barriers of politics, culture, gender and ethnicity. Our identities are fragmentary and constantly in the process of being remade, which is both challenging and a possibility for creativity (Weeks, 1995, pp. 85–6).

In pursuing the analysis of individual and social dimensions of the experiences of AIDS in later chapters, this contemporary theorization of society will provide the bedrock for interpreting the local meanings of AIDS in relation to different forms of identity. In the final chapter I bring together material on how sexual identities may be changing and how AIDS is changing to suggest how their intersection may be in flux at century's end.

The idea of critical communities points to one feature of identities which is at the heart of my analysis. In this perspective identity is a reflexive project. In other words, we all build our identities out of a number of existing fragments, be they of class, gender, race, religion, sexuality and so forth. As members of critical communities we shape these elements in what may be original directions, as in 'am I queer rather than gay, and what does this mean?' A clear implication of all this is that identity is something which has to be achieved; it is not given in tradition. Not only is it to be achieved, it has no end point. In late modernity we are faced with having constantly to fashion our identities, to pursue our life narratives. If we accept this perspective, a clear implication is that contemporary identities are better understood in terms of processes than essences or structured positions within society and culture. Identity is in a sense something that someone performs as much as what they are.

In the next chapter this idea of identity as process forms the basis of explaining my perspective on what identity is (a theoretical position), and how it can be investigated (the appropriate methodology). In doing this I am not attempting a wide-ranging review of the social science literature on identity, but pointing to the utility of a particular approach in exploring my wider theme of the intersection of identities and AIDS in 1990s Britain.

Note

1. I don't intend a thorough description of the history of identity politics connected with sexuality here. The history is well documented in sources such as Weeks, 1985 and 1995, and current theoretical debates in sociology and cultural studies can be found, for example, in Seidman, 1996.

2

Identities in Perspective

The subject of identity, as suggested in Chapter 1, is at the forefront of contemporary social science, particularly as it engages with the nature of late modernity in Western society. Across the spectrum of the social sciences the frame of reference for viewing identity varies, and within any discipline's perspective interests change over time. At one end of the spectrum, psychology is interested in identity as an expression of individual disposition, grounded in genetics and shaped most strongly by familial socialization. In this view, identities are gained through childhood, but in general, the adult identity of a person is seen as a fairly stable entity. Identity may later change as a result of trauma, most notably where the brain is damaged physically. For psychologists our identities shape our social interactions, and are logically prior to them. In behavioural psychology, individual personality or identity traits can be tested experimentally.

At the other end of the social science spectrum, anthropology and interpretive sociology, working with the organizing concepts of culture and society, are more interested in the ways in which identities are shaped at group level and, just as importantly, how culturally and societally specific ideas about what identity is shape our experience of our identities. In other words, they are interested in identity as a social product more than as an expression of individual psychological dispositions.

This division of focus is in one sense arbitrary. Genetics sets the boundaries to individual potentials, and early socialization clearly has profound impacts on our personalities and senses of self. Yet those selves are acted out in social and cultural contexts, and our understandings and evaluation of the self are shaped by the circulation of ideas in our social circles and wider culture (for example, there are well-known cultural stereotypes about the desirability or otherwise of certain personality traits). Psychology and the more 'social' social sciences can be seen as each contributing to the broader picture of what identity is. This is to suggest a complementary rather than antagonistic set of perspectives, ignoring some more fundamental differences of opinion. To review extensively the literature on identity and how it has developed in different academic disciplines is a large task and one I won't attempt here. I will be taking a particular line on what identity is and how to investigate it, but this first needs some justification in relation to competing perspectives.

The self as essence

In spite of all the social science of recent years, the belief that we have a true inner and immutable self remains powerful in Western cultures. This view is nurtured both by belief in transcendent religion (we have unique souls which need saving) and transcendent science (we are unique constellations of genetic material to be transferred, rearranged, in perpetuity). This latter view has become popularized especially since the publication in 1976 of zoologist Richard Dawkins' *The Selfish Gene*, which retheorizes evolution as being about the successful transmission of genetic material through time. The historical nature of these beliefs is explored in Foucault's later work on the history of sexuality, in which he traces the development of a preoccupation with locating the truth of the self in the sexualized body (Foucault, 1978). His analysis draws attention simultaneously to the development of ideas about sexuality from the religious to the medical and the ways in which these changes made possible new subjectivities, in other words that people came to have identities premised on sexuality, which had not previously been possible. Foucault locates these emergent identities in the nineteenth century. Later writers have proposed earlier dates, drawing on specific historical records, but are in agreement that sexual identities with which we are familiar in the West emerged at an identifiable period in history, in the context of secularization, the rise of science and medicine, and attendant changes in laws relating to sexual conduct (e.g. Weeks, 1981; Halperin,

1990). The key figure in all of this was the homosexual, a recognized kind of person who did not exist before. Foucault and other writers all recognized that same-gender sexual desires are in all probability trans-historical (and in some senses transcultural) but that the idea of the homosexual as a person with a distinct way of life, and indeed a self-conception of being a homosexual, was an historical novelty. In other words, a homosexual identity is something historically and socially constructed, not the expression of some inner essence (whether this is assumed to be God-given or genetically determined). I will return to the theme of social constructionism in presenting my own perspective, but for now wish to enlarge on Foucault's noting of the emergence of certain kinds of essentialized identities.

The truth about the self is revealed through confession. In Western society Christian religions have demanded the truth from the individual, the revelation of and repentance for sins, most notably in the Roman Catholic confessional. What Foucault says is that confessing did not disappear with secularization. If anything, it became augmented, though it was directed elsewhere. The confessional moved from the church to the psychoanalyst's and psychiatrist's couches. In both psychoanalysis and psychiatry the self came to be identified with a sexualized self, one that underwent a process of development which could be successful or incomplete and pathological. In Freudian psychoanalysis this process was identified with the resolution (or failed resolution) of the Oedipal conflict. If the resolution was unsuccessful, neurosis was the result, and adult homosexuality one possible variety of neurosis (though Freud's views on homosexuality were subtle and contradictory). All this suggests that nurture plays a role in the development of the self as well as nature, allowing a rapprochement between psychoanalysis and social constructionist perspectives; indeed contemporary social scientists are re-evaluating Freud as a key to linking cultural processes and the development of individual subjectivity (see Moore, 1994). But Foucault's point was that at the time of the rise of psychoanalysis and psychiatry, the therapeutic process focused on confession. The presenting problems of the patient were an expression of hidden inner conflict (the repressed in Freudian terms). The purpose of the therapist was to help the patient uncover the hidden inner self, which required the patient to confess the most intimate details of his or her inner and outer lives.

The process of analysis assumed a hidden inner self (the unconscious), something at the core of the person, and though subject to shaping (notably through relationships with parents), this idea of a hidden inner truth continued an essentialist idea of identity. Foucault is saying that the various psychotherapies and psychiatry (as well as, as I have suggested, psychology) have an inherently essentialist conception of identity. More importantly, though, he is arguing that their models of identity were themselves historical products, not the triumph of rational science. The conditions for the possibility of a certain understanding of human nature and identity only arose during the nineteenth century, but these understandings have been refined and remain extremely powerful in the knowledges of biomedicine, psychotherapy and psychiatry.

The historical construction of identities

The view that certain identities did, and could only, emerge in specific historic circumstances, is most closely associated with Foucault's work. Many other scholars have taken up his framework in looking at the historical rise of sexual identities in the West, either broadly in agreement (Weeks, 1985; Halperin, 1990, 1997) or to argue against him for the transhistorical nature of sexual identities (Boswell, 1980). All these analyses look at the construction of identities in relatively great historical depth. Elsewhere in the social sciences constructionist perspectives are applied to identity, but in shorter time frames. The analyses of sociologists and anthropologists, except in the case of longitudinal studies, tend to be synchronic in focus, though the best of them take account of historical context as well.

Anthropology, with its focus on culture, chiefly non-Western culture, is interested in the different ways in which cultures organize their ideas about the social world and how to act in it. Interpretive sociology does similar things, but more often in First World societies. Both disciplines work from the assumption that cultural and social ideas are creative projects that can take many forms, but can usually be interpreted as bearing inherent logics that can be investigated (otherwise anthropology and sociology would be a waste of time). They consider that the social and the cultural are levels and forms of explanation with a distinct ontological status. They do not accept that all social and cultural phenomena can be reduced to biological imperatives. So they would strongly take issue with some of the claims of sociobiology that all human behaviour can be explained as an expression of the evolutionary principle of natural selection. This is not to deny that genetics has connections with social and cultural phenomena, but rather to say that the arguments of some branches of natural science are crudely reductionist and teleological. But the argument is more sophisticated than this. Contemporary anthropology and interpretive sociology tend to the view, not that there are natural laws of society (as early sociologists such as Durkheim held) but that the social and the cultural, in line more widely with late modernist and postmodernist thought, have to be understood as reflexive products of human consciousness. In other words, culture and society do not have an objective existence independent of the social actors who constitute them. Culture and society are always already inventions and interpretations, or (as Judith Butler notably says) performances (Butler, 1989, 1993). If we accept this (admittedly contentious) view, then objectivist and positivist analyses of culture and society have no inherent status; they become one invention, or construction, among others.

This brief sketch of contemporary theoretical concerns in anthropology and sociology provides one rationale for looking at identities as being socially constructed: they must be as much what we decide they are in particular cultural and historical circumstances as they are 'things' in their own right, even leaving aside the possibility that race, gender and, just possibly, sexual orientation (if one accepts 'gay gene' or 'gay hypothalamus' theories) have a biological substrate not easily amenable to cultural manipulation. Yet there is a simpler reason for accepting that identities may be constructions. The ethnographic record shows that various aspects of persons are considered very differently in different cultural settings. To take an example pertinent here, the apparent incidence of homosexual behaviours, how they are regarded, and the senses in which they are associated with particular identities are highly culturally variable. A literature on the cultural construction of sexuality is growing within anthropology, which locates particular behaviours and identities in the wider cultural contexts of ideas about reproduction, kinship, the family and political control over biological and social reproduction. It situates analysis of sexuality within what have been termed sex–gender systems (Ortner and Whitehead, 1981, introduction) and provides evidence that attitudes to sexuality when considered comparatively reflect cultural ideologies about gender and the appropriate roles of men and women, masculinity and femininity, in society.

To illustrate variations in cultural constructions of sexuality, and the need to conceptualize sexuality in broader cultural fields, we can turn to Melanesian ethnography, specifically to studies of certain hill tribes of Papua New Guinea. This literature, particularly the work of Gilbert Herdt, problematizes the relationship between sexual behaviours, identities and the nature of desire (Herdt, 1983). It even raises problems about the category 'sexuality' itself.

The Sambia, Etoro, Marind-anim, Kiwai and other hill peoples have practised initiation rites that mark the passage from childhood to adulthood. In this they are like many other non-Western societies that anthropologists have observed to mark transitions between life stages through rites of passage. These practices are largely dying out now: for reasons that will become apparent, Christian influence has discouraged them, though they persist to some extent, for example among the Sambia (as recorded in *Guardian of the Flutes* for the Channel Four series *Under the Sun*).

The rites apply only to boys. In local conceptions of adulthood, the onset of menstruation marks the beginning of womanhood. No such naturally occurring boundary marker is recognized for boys, though. Instead, cultural practices mark and reinforce a transition from boy to man. At about the age of ten, boys are separated from their parental houses and sent to live with other initiates in long-houses separate from the villages. They remain here through adolescence, and are initiated into male adulthood by those who have already passed through the rituals. The rituals are diverse, and include teaching about warriorhood and the adult role. They culminate in the secret knowledge of the flutes, which are blown during the more clandestine rituals, and represent the penis. In the way that the elders blow the flutes, so the initiates must suck the penises of their elders.

What is this all about? In Sambia terms, as interpreted by Herdt, boys lack semen, which is thought symbolically and actually to be the locus of male power (and is symbolically equivalent to menstrual blood for women). Boys become transformed into men by ingesting the semen of their elders and, once past puberty, in their turn inseminate the younger initiates.

Taken out of context, these behaviours would be labelled by a Westerner as homosexual: they are sexual because they involve physical stimulation to orgasm, and homosexual because they involve persons of the same sex. Yet Herdt cautions against such a reading. At least in the past, these practices involved a majority of Sambia boys, most of whom in adult life married and had no further same-sex sexual contact. The behaviour seemed to have no link to a sexual identity in the way we might expect in the West. Further, the process of insemination was thought to masculinize the boys, whereas in most European and North American contexts being penetrated by another man is considered unmanning and feminizing. Instead, Herdt asks us to understand this cultural complex as being about an ideology of appropriate gender roles and relations, and that the initiation rituals reflect and reinforce a hegemonic heterosexual order, rather than encourage difference. Sambian society is highly sex-segregated, with men as top dogs. The initiations make men of boys, after which time they return to society to become fathers, while maintaining a dominant political association with other men. The symbolism of semen versus menstrual blood is always relational, with male symbols superior to female, but potentially threatened by them. In this analysis, the activities in the initiation rites are perhaps not best seen as primarily sexual.

This focus on wider sets of culturally specific values is a valuable addition to our understanding of sexuality and gender, but contains its own problems. The cultural focus of anthropology tends to evade the embodied aspects of sexuality. The gap in analysis has reflected a certain squeamishness (personal and professional) among anthropologists about investigating 'private' sexual behaviours. In whatever ways sexuality is constructed, at some level it is linked with the physical and emotional responses of the human body. Anthropology has steered around this linkage because sexuality has tended to be seen in individualistic and psychological terms, aspects of the person which anthropologists tend to treat as anterior to culture, and properly the domain of individualistic sciences such as psychology. Anthropologists would say they are not so much interested in the acquisition of individuality as in such questions as 'what constitutes the idea of individuality in a given cultural context'. As Henrietta Moore argues in *A Passion for Difference* (1994, ch. 2) this is question begging since it leaves untheorized any link between individual and group self-consciousness. To fill this gap, anthropologists are beginning to turn to psychoanalytical theory, since Freud provides a possible key for linking individual and collective consciousness without falling a priori into the traps of methodological individualism or methodological collectivism (Born, 1994).

It is this direction that Gilbert Herdt has taken in refining his analysis of Sambia sexual ideology to take account of the embodied nature of the rituals, and individuals whose social positions appear anomalous in relation to collective practices. In *Intimate Communications: Erotics and the Study of Culture* (1990) he teamed up with Robert Stoller, a psychoanalyst, to revisit his Sambia communities and look at individual experiences and life histories in relation to the male initiation rites. Interviews explored the physical aspects of the rites as well as their cultural meanings. Many respondents had found them painful or unpleasant, and were quite content to practise sexually only within marriage thereafter. Their personal sexual inclinations went against what the cultural rituals prescribed. Yet there were a few men for whom the experiences had different implications. These individuals, regarded by others as eccentrics, did not marry as adults and continued only to have oral sexual contact as the inseminators of boys. Herdt and Stoller concluded that these individuals more nearly approximated what would be called homosexual in Western terms, in that they seemed to have a preference for same-sex erotic object choice, which ran counter to cultural expectations (Herdt and Stoller, 1990, ch. 9). Yet Herdt and Stoller maintain the need for a carefully considered constructionism. These unusual individuals had experienced oral sex with other boys just like their 'conventional' age-mates. Without further research it would be difficult to identify a single cause for their adult propensity (was it nature, or nurture, or both?). Furthermore, their sexual interests could not be said to relate to a recognizable identity based on sexual difference, such as being gay in the West. At most they were just thought of as unusual, and since others had shared their sexual practices they were not labelled with such strong terms as deviance or dissidence.

Herdt and Stoller's analysis points to the need to consider carefully the intersection of cultural values and personal experience in trying to map the intersections of sexual behaviours, sexuality and identities. Their joint analyses go beyond a difficulty in Herdt's earlier work, that the culturalist interpretations of the initiation rituals call into question the category sexuality itself. If the activities recorded do not 'mean' something in terms of erotic choice then we have the problem that genital sexuality is not everywhere accorded sexual status, which is counter-intuitive in terms of what is known about the physiology of sexual arousal. We run the risk of a total cultural relativism in which the body is only a cultural artefact. *Intimate Communications* gets around this problem by suggesting that the narratives of 'unconventional' individuals reflect the embodied nature of the ritual experiences, since these experiences carry over into adult sexual preferences. And in a commonsense vein, Carol Vance, quoting a student posed with the question of whether we can *assume* these ritual activities to be sexual, says of these Papua New Guineans that 'Their cosmology posits that young boys grow to adulthood only through the ingestion of semen, but you don't see them eating it with a bowl and spoon' (Vance, 1989, p. 22). These arguments suggest that culture plays a major role in defining what is sexual and how it is experienced, but that the biological workings of the body put limits to these definitions, limits which are transcultural.

The position that Herdt and Stoller take to reconcile constructionism with the body can be described as middle-ground constructionism (Vance, 1989, p.19). In the debate between essentialist and constructionist positions on identity it is vital to distinguish a number of degrees of constructionism. All constructionist social scientists interested in sexuality take the view that any given item of sexual behaviour can vary in its meaning cross-culturally, and that the relationship between sexual behaviours and identities is therefore fluid. Beyond this, the idea of a sexual community, and how individuals belong to such communities, also varies. This is the middle-ground view reflected by Herdt and Stoller. A more radical variant of constructionism argues that the direction of sexual object choice (sexual orientation) is constructed and not an inherent genetic/biological aspect of the individual. This is the source of much contestation between essentialists and constructionists about homosexuality in the West. The essentialists (a label I am applying: few would deliberately label themselves essentialist) now argue that male homosexuality is caused by an identifiable gene (Toufexis, 1995) and that there are brain differences between heterosexual and homosexual men. Middle-ground constructionists would argue that there *may* be a biological influence on sexual orientation, but that it is not a sufficient cause for adult orientation and sexual identity, and that these are highly culturally variable. The more radical constructionists argue that biology has nothing to do with it: sexual orientation and identity are entirely historical, social and cultural products. In its most extreme form constructionism considers the very category 'sexual' to be invalid as a universal human term. This position has relatively few adherents, given that most of the evidence suggests that throughout cultures there is an area of life that can reasonably be termed sexual without too much distortion through translation.

Making these distinctions among levels of constructionism is important to advancing my perspective on identity. I am taking a middle-ground constructionist perspective. That is to say, that some aspects of an identity may be laid down prior to social and cultural influence, but that the latter are of great importance (and that this may apply to aspects of identity other than sexuality). Some fundamental aspects of personality may be laid down genetically, but this cannot account for the working out of identities through the life course.

Analytic time frames

These are theoretical concerns influencing how identity is thought about. Another concern, which links theory with methodology, is central to the position I am adopting: time frames. In the studies discussed so far, the picturing of identity is generally through retrospective accounts of individual life histories. In other words, they are historical analyses in a narrow sense. Other perspectives on identity in contemporary social and anthropological theory point to the interactive nature of culture, the aspect of constructionism which focuses on culture as invention and performance (and the general thrust of contemporary social theory, discussed in Chapter 1, which suggests that we increasingly have to invent ourselves). To add these dimensions, at least in empirical research, implies that we need to be there while it is happening. Identity is the accretion of a number of performances throughout the life cycle. One kind of study that can contribute pieces of the picture, therefore, is one that draws on observation in naturally occurring social situations as well as personal reflections in interviews, contemporary and retrospective. It is these varieties of empirical data that are drawn on in this book.

Pursuing the methodological implications of recent theoretical positions on identity, and particularly the interactive aspects of identity formation, Ken Plummer's *Telling Sexual Stories* (1995) argues that the reflexive project of the self in contemporary Western society is realized in large part through stories we tell about ourselves. We construct narratives about ourselves and our histories that explain to ourselves and those connected with us socially and culturally who we are. In the late modern

West these stories focus on the sexualized self. Thus, a paradigmatic sexual story is the 'coming out' story of the gay man, lesbian, or bisexual. It is a story of becoming and accepting a stigmatized identity (Blasius, 1994). Plummer characterizes sexual stories in terms of individual and social consequence, and requires a number of related questions to be posed of them:

- *What is the nature of a story?* How do we classify a story in the literary sense of genre and trope? What narrative form does the story take?
- *What are the social processes of producing and consuming a story?* How do people come to produce a story? What might silence them? Who hears a story, under what circumstances, and how is it heard in relation to the social world in which it is constructed?
- *What are the social roles that a story plays?* Once a story is told, what wider function might it have in promoting or inhibiting interests in a political context? How does the confessional content of a story inflect wider cultural concerns?
- *What is the role of change, history and culture?* Following Foucault, what makes it possible for certain stories to be told by certain people, and heard and responded to by certain others, at some points of time and place but not others?
 (Plummer, 1995, pp. 24–5)

Plummer is indicating the need to see stories as an important aspect of identities, which must be situated in the interaction of a number of different levels and processes. In this he is continuing the tradition of symbolic interactionism in sociology, which sees social and cultural phenomena as lying in the production and circulation of shared symbols, a process that results from social interaction, and is not in any sense prior to or programmed into social interaction as essentialist perspectives might argue.

Symbolic interactionist assumptions inform the constructionist perspective of this book, but its methodological premises are slightly different from Plummer's. The specific stories he quotes are either stories published by individuals or elicited from them in research. They are for the most part reflective written accounts of some length, and published in written format and are therefore public documents. This is an important channel through which stories get told, but I would argue it is only one aspect of the telling of sexual (and other) stories. The symbolic inter-actionist perspective is about interaction and performance as well as the written word. We live in a literate culture in which reading is prominent, yet stories get told in our everyday interactions as well. This suggests that research into telling stories needs to include these everyday interactions as well as printed stories (and, now, stories on the Internet). At the same time, some form of observation and interaction by a researcher might lead to different accounts, for example, of how a particular story came to be told, and to a particular audience, than what the author of the story might relate in a retrospective, written account. Participant observation, and interviewing guided by observation, may enrich a study of story-telling otherwise reliant only on published stories.

A second point implicit in a social interactionist and constructionist perspective is that if identity is a performance, and story-telling is a delimited field of performance, though we may accept that 'telling sexual stories' is a key feature of the formation of contemporary identities in the West, it can never offer an exhaustive account of identities. Other ways in which we come to reflect on ourselves in interaction with others need exploring.

Limitations in constructionist and interactionist methodologies

Before explaining exactly how the empirical data represented in this book were collected in pursuit of a constructionist perspective on identity, it is necessary to discuss critically limitations to this kind of perspective. These limitations concern the status of identity in constructionist accounts, whose identities we are discussing and the utility of the concept of identity itself.

I have so far promoted an understanding of identity grounded in symbolic interactionism. One main criticism of this approach appeals to common sense. Whether essential or constructed, in the West we all possess a very strong sense of a self and a unique identity. The problem with the symbolic interactionist model of the self is that it ends up being too contingent and fluctuating: there is no adequate explanation for such strong senses of self developing. It is also weak in explaining the relation between the individual self and the group self (Cohen, 1994, p. 11). Cohen, proposing an alternative anthropology of identity, argues for a

32

modification of symbolic interactionism. He holds that the term 'symbol' should be used in the sense of a vehicle for interpretation, not as a literal referent to something else. A symbol can at one level connote something recognizable to all members of a community, yet at another level hold more idiosyncratic meanings for individuals (*ibid.*, p. 18). This perspective allows for apparent agreement at group level while also accounting for greater conflict in interpretation between individuals. It preserves individuality among group identities while still being a constructionist perspective. As an example, Cohen, citing Stromberg, refers to the relationship between individual religious believers and the dogmatic symbols of organized religion. Among Pietists in Stockholm apparently shared theology and religious dogmas are used to make entirely personal commitments to the faith, and the individualization of belief and practice is a defining feature of Pietism. The religion offers common forms of worship and a congregation; yet these forms are relatively insubstantial. Pietists are explicitly invited to give meaning to these forms through their personal experience of their faith so that

> people may share commitments without sharing beliefs; it follows that they may constitute a community without that community being based in consensus. (Stromberg, 1986, p. 13)

and

> common discourse is forged out of diverse meanings rather than shared ones. (*ibid.*, p. 51)

The implications of Cohen's arguments are that the individual and collective levels have to be understood as implicating each other, and that symbolic forms have to be interrogated individually and collectively in a number of settings in order to be understood. Methodologically speaking, studies of identity must address all of these to produce a coherent and complete picture. Further, since the interpretation of symbols involves particular individuals in relation to identifiable groups, the meanings attached, say, to particular kinds of identity can vary highly according to context; identities, then, will always be moving targets. The common forms and idiosyncratic interpretations must be distinguished, otherwise we may end in the twin traps of methodological universalism or methodological individualism.

A second, related, criticism of symbolic interactionist approaches is that they mistake identity for the performance of identity. In this view, although the life course modifies identity, if we look at discrete episodes of social interaction, all we are observing is the acting out of pre-existing identities. What people say and do is premised on the identities they carry around with them. This is a possibly valid criticism of the empirical data presented in this book. Timescale of data collection does matter, and it is difficult to write exhaustive accounts of identity based on small fragments of life. On these lines I will try to make the claims for the empirical data modest. The counter-argument to this is that a rigid distinction between identities and their performance in social context is implicitly essentialist. Over time, it can be argued, the effect of acting out identities in interaction with others is that the sense of self may change, and this in turn may affect future interactions. If not, we are left with the self as a kind of private residue of the social and, following Cohen's logic, no way of reconciling personal and group senses of identity.

A third limitation lies in the inadequacies of constructionism in general, of which symbolic interactionism is one species. Some of these relate to an overreliance on the category 'identity'. Hening Bech elaborates this point in suggesting that the concept of gay identity under-theorizes all men's connections with culturally validated forms of masculinity, and relations between non-homosexual men and homosexuality (Bech, 1997, pp. 2ff); I discuss these ideas in greater detail in Chapter 6. Steven Epstein proposes that in practice 'identity' as an analytic category tends towards either psychological or sociological reductionism (Epstein, 1987, p. 144). In other words it is either used psychologically to refer to an unfolding of an inner self (a definition that is individualistic and essentialist) or sociologically, in which case identity is merely what the group agrees it to be and, therefore, experiences it to be. The sociological end of the continuum is also associated with constructionism, and Epstein takes some variants of constructionism to task for implying that identity is something we can endlessly fashion in limitless ways. An appeal to common sense and the empirical evidence obviously contradicts such total relativism. These criticisms are rather like Cohen's: the relations between an idiosyncratic personal identity and social and cultural values through which identity can be apprehended and developed cannot be theorized using diametrically opposed conceptions of identity and unconstrained constructionism. Epstein's answer to this is to invoke Habermas' notion of 'ego identity' (Habermas, 1979), and to suggest that there are external limitations on identity construction (discursive, ideological, political, economic) so that people can (paraphrasing Marx) make their identities, but not exactly as they please.

> Ego identity, then, is a *socialized sense of identity*, an internal organization of self-perceptions concerning one's relationship to social categories, that also incorporates views of the self perceived to be held by others. (Epstein, 1987, p. 19)

In this view sexual identity, class, gender and race identity are subsidiary to ego identity. This fits with the perspective developed here, which is that identities are shifting mosaics of competing elements. What is not clear from Habermas' formulation is how the relative importance of these elements comes about, and changes, or how the external constraints on identity construction operate. In much of this book, gay identities are both strongly felt and strongly articulated, though they do not exhaust the identity of any individual. My argument is that context becomes a crucial element. I will be demonstrating how identities are performed in contexts that shape them. In this case, for most of the time, the contexts are HIV/AIDS voluntary sector organizations and the people involved in them. In doing this my analysis leans towards a sociologically rather than psychologically biased definition of identity. I will be indicating how political and other forces delimit the possibilities of identity choice, but more in terms of group identity performance than individual self-consciousness. This is not, then, an exhaustive account of the relations between individual and group in identity terms (and I only make use of a few group examples); nor do I offer a sophisticated neo-Foucauldian analysis of the discursive determinants of identity.

Whose identities?

My discussion so far has focused on debates about sexual identities, justified by the centrality of sexuality in Western conceptions of the self. But this book is about identities in the context of AIDS, and sexuality does not exhaust the identities of everyone affected by AIDS (and the question is begged of whether the identities even of sexual minorities such as gay men are exhausted by sexuality). An apologist response might be that contemporary politics in the West is increasingly a politics of identity and new social movements, and that identity is premised on lifestyle (Plummer, 1995; Giddens, 1991, 1992; Weeks, 1995). These considerations are coming to replace earlier forms of identification based on social divisions of race, ethnicity, gender and class. The problem with this argument is that these very social divisions in varying degrees do still play important roles in people's senses of self and social belonging. If we are to look at women with AIDS, ethnic minority men and women, and heterosexual injecting drugs users, we must adopt a methodology that does not foreground sexuality at the expense of other relevant aspects of identity.

Identity as analytic concept: further comments

An exploration of the history of lesbian and gay politics by Mark Blasius calls into question the usefulness of applying the term identity to the experiences of lesbians and gay men. He proposes that the combination of a sexual orientation, a differentiated lifestyle and a sense of community linked with lifestyle is best analysed in terms of a concept of *ethos* rather than identity. The fact that sexuality is of primary importance in the West, but a problem for lesbians and gay men, provides an impetus for community formation among lesbians and gay men (Blasius, 1994, p. 6). In this community formation Blasius sees possibilities for the integration of friendship and sexuality, a kind of erotically informed ideology, which is not available to the heterosexual mainstream. Clearly some same-sex identified individuals participate much more in community than do others (some do not at all), though we all belong to a subculture of which we are aware by virtue of our sexual behaviours.

Blasius sees 'ethos' as a more encompassing term than orientation or lifestyle, while it also goes beyond the limitations of seeing lesbian and gay life primarily in terms of subculture or community. It does refer to an explicit sense of being lesbian or gay, not just sexual behaviour devoid of identity referents, but an individual can participate in this ethos at a number of levels. The rationale for thinking in terms of ethos is that being lesbian or gay depends on the process of coming out, which means embracing a stigmatized, political identity. This begins with self-realization of being lesbian or gay, and goes on to public avowal in various contexts, a process that may continue for the rest of the life cycle. Coming out is a process of becoming a lesbian or gay man, of collectively problematizing the self (*ibid.*, p. 180). Out of a sense of difference and minority status is forged an ethos of searching for a lesbian and gay 'communitas', an ideal type community and sense of belonging. Blasius sees lesbian and gay ethos as being productive of knowledge and truths of existence as seen from lesbian and gay perspectives. Ethos is the site of production of a distinctive lesbian and gay discourse of life.

Should we, then, abandon identity and think instead in terms of ethos? If our subject is broader than a debate about contemporary lesbian and gay identities then there are good reasons not to abandon identity altogether. Blasius develops his notion of ethos carefully in relation to lesbians and gay men, and it is not clear whether it would be relevant to other groups. Becoming a woman or a black British person does not involve a 'coming out' process or identification with others over something premised on lifestyle. Secondly, as I have already illustrated, the late modern world in the West is saturated with discussion of identity. Paraphrasing Carole Vance's argument about the ultimate construction-ist abandoning of the concept 'sexuality', it is counter-intuitive to reject altogether the concept of identity as an analytic tool. To retain it, though, means taking care to be very precise in use of the term, since it can be used to make fundamentally incompatible arguments. Like 'community', 'identity' can be a weasel word.

Identity and research methods: a specific approach

The perspective I am pursuing is one in which identities are built through the acquisition of culturally shared symbols, but, in line with Cohen, symbols whose precise significance can be idiosyncratically interpreted and manipulated by the individual. At the same time, identities are always in a process of becoming and contain a performative dimension. In line with contemporary social theory, I hold that contemporary identities in the West are shifting mosaics (Gatter, 1995). Identities have to be created by us, and consist of overlapping and sometimes competing elements, of gender, sexuality, ethnicity, class, age, geographical region and other factors. Identities are dialectical and which particular aspects of a complex identity are uppermost shift with history and context. The thrust of analyses of late modernity is that sexual identities will occupy a privileged position among other forms of identification, but be in dialectical relationship with them.

A complete account of an individual's identity therefore implies an unrealistic task: the collection of personal, reflective narratives (as in Plummer's work) and observation, over a considerable period, of the person in his or her varied contexts of social interaction. Research into identity within the proposed theoretical framing has necessarily to be selective and partial.

The empirical data presented and interpreted in this book are of two kinds. First, there are notes based on participant observation in an AIDS Service Organization (ASO). These notes cover a wide range of aspects of the 'life' of this organization as seen from the researcher's perspective. They include conversations between people at the Centre[1] (users of Centre services, volunteers and staff), group discussions, and conversations with me. Out of this 'stream' of data I have excerpted examples of people behaving as part of identifiable groups, and overtly discussing issues from identity perspectives: as gay men, as women, as Black, and so on, and use these to develop arguments about individual and group identity in Chapters 3 and 4. The second kind of data were collected through semi-structured interviews with individuals. In these interviews people were invited to describe their personal histories of living with HIV before being asked more specific questions about their use and experience of HIV/AIDS services. The interviews generated 'stories' of living with HIV in Plummer's sense, though these were stories told to an individual who was known by the narrator to be evaluating the services of the centre at which the interviews were conducted.

These kinds of data broadly reflect the research traditions of anthropology. As anthropologists, we assume that the life worlds of our research subjects may be very different from our own (a necessary assumption, perhaps, where non-literate, non-Western cultures are the subject of research). We therefore aim to build an interpretation of these life worlds through careful inductive reasoning. We try to build a picture of what, for example, sexuality 'means' in a given cultural context by looking for characteristic patterns of thought in a much broader set of cultural symbols. The general aim of this approach is avoidance of imposing predetermined hypotheses. Also, the voices of our research subjects should come across without being lost in excessively general abstractions. Such an approach is complementary to the problem of identity. As argued, Western thinking on and experience of identity are heavily predicated on sexuality. Yet we know that identity is made up of other elements as well. A non-directive, inductive and qualitative approach to research potentially allows these various identity factors to emerge through the data.

This aside, the bulk of the analysis in this book concerns sexuality. Without apology, this is connected to the author's interests and the fact that a great deal of the current literature on identity concerns sexuality, particularly homosexuality. In Britain gay men as a group are disproportionately affected by HIV, and the majority of respondents in our research, both in participant observation and interviews, were gay men. Methodologically speaking, my own subject position as a gay man was significant. In participant observation it soon became clear that those around me assumed where I 'fitted in'. In interviews with other gay men the sense of something shared was productive in terms of trust and rapport. With interviewees who were not gay men the opposite could apply: the narrative of the interview might be shaped by the perception of the interviewee that I shared a perspective with a group of people to which the interviewee did not belong. There is, however, a methodological conundrum here, because the effects of identification with interviewees can be reversed (for example, a gay man finding it easier to talk openly to someone perceived as less linked to the self, or a woman feeling uncomfortable talking to an interviewer perceived as a heterosexual man). There is no certainty or methodological prescription, though the general recommendation is that some implicit identification between researcher and subject is generally productive, with the caveat that over-identification can lead to loss of objectivity or, as it was politically incorrectly called in anthropology, 'going native' (see Ellen, 1984; Pelto and Pelto, 1978; Hammersley, 1992). Practically, I decided not to disclose my sexuality in interview unless asked explicitly. To have done so might have shaped too strongly the nature of interaction in the interview. On the other hand, disclosure occurs by means other than overt declaration: interviewees may have made inferences about who and what I was (accurate or otherwise) based on dress, behaviour, body language and the content of conversations that bracketed the interviews. Such matters are beyond strict methodological control.

The data collected through participant observation and interviews cannot be used to make claims about identity over the life course. The interviews do, though, give some time depth to the observation of the 'performance' of identity in 'real time'. Care is needed, however, in assuming that interview and observation data have the same status, or that interview data automatically support observational data, and we cannot assess the latter unless both sets of data refer to the same individual and the same events (what is methodologically termed data triangulation).

The immediacy of the observation data, and the fact that interviewees reflected on events at the Centre during the period of the evaluation, mean that relatively strong arguments can be made about the performative aspects of identity. It is possible to elaborate on shared identity symbols, their more personal and idiosyncratic meanings and how symbols were contested in a setting in which different groups competed for limited resources (some services were always at a premium in the Centre). It can also be argued that these contests become some of the material through which individuals understand themselves, and therefore shape their identities.

As well as primary data from my empirical research, I use secondary data that make arguments about identity in relation to HIV and AIDS. Thus I examine the proclamations of groups such as Gay Men Fighting AIDS (GMFA), who have an explicit aim to promote gay men's interests around HIV/AIDS. This secondary material I use to complement the primary analysis, particularly when I examine claims about identity and community in Chapter 4. My purpose in using this data is to examine how claims about identity and community are made by individuals who play a relatively powerful role in shaping the 'gay discourse' of AIDS in Britain.

The context of the research

The data that I describe are drawn from a larger piece of research which also involved Rayah Feldman at South Bank University and Andrew Bebbington and Pat Warren of the University of Kent. This evaluation of an HIV/AIDS social care voluntary organization in inner London was funded by the Department of Health. The evaluation ran from Autumn 1989 until June 1992. The purpose of the evaluation was to assess the Centre as an innovatory model for a range of care services housed in one building. To do this, a complex, four-strand research programme was devised with the following aims:

- Statistical analysis of the use of Centre services, in comparison with other ASOs.
- Study of the development of the Centre in terms of its policies and management structure.
- Study of the impact of the setting up of the Centre on other providers in the HIV/AIDS sector.
- Study of the direct impact of the Centre on the lives of its service users.

My role in this was the fourth strand, the direct impact study. This was to be done via interviews with service users, but I added participant observation as an extra source of data. As a means to becoming integrated at the Centre for participant observation, and to make a practical contribution during the research, I also opted to train and work as a volunteer, and continued in this role between June 1990 and June 1992.

The Centre consisted of a central social drop-in area, shared by service users, staff and volunteers, together with other shared facilities such as a library and laundry, and private rooms for one-to-one service sessions. These latter ranged from money advice and social work to complementary therapies (including reflexology, shiatsu, Swedish massage and homoeopathy). Much of the observation data were collected while working as a volunteer around the drop-in area, though weekly staff meetings and monthly meetings of the board of directors were also attended. Written notes were taken in meetings, but not within the drop-in or at volunteer meetings (by mutual agreement) as this would have seemed intrusive and surveillant. I would write up the events of the day after leaving the Centre, or in privacy while there. My role as evaluator was made known to all at the Centre, and reiterated during the period of research.

I conducted interviews with 46 service users, 34 of whom I reinterviewed approximately one year later to review their interim experiences.[2] These interviewees were diverse according to age, gender, sexuality, route of transmission of HIV and time since HIV-positive diagnosis (see Table 2.1).

The interviews began by recording some basic demographic data, and then asked the interviewee to describe his or her experience of living with HIV, which led interviewees to describe the circumstances and experience of testing positive. After this, more specific questions were posed about

Table 2.1: Interviewee characteristics

Characteristic	Number	Percentage
Gender		
Male	45	78
Female	13	22
HIV transmission route		
Sex between men	37	64
Heterosexual sex	10	17
Needle-sharing	7	12
Other	1	2
Untested	3	5
Social class (ONS)[3]		
I	13	22
II	8	14
IIIN	11	19
IIIM	8	14
IV	9	16
V	6	10
Unclassified	3	5
Ethnicity		
White British/Irish	44	76
Black British/Afro-Caribbean	3	5
Black African	3	5
European	7	12
Latin American	1	2
Time since diagnosis		
Less than 1 year	16	28
More than 1 year	39	67
Untested	3	5
Centre service use		
User	47	81
Non-user	11	19

experiences of health and social services, use of voluntary organizations, and finally how the interviewees had come to use the Centre, what services they used, and what benefits they experienced. They were also questioned on their social experience of the Centre and their interaction with and attitudes towards other service users.

In sum, this was applied research with the specific goal of assessing critically the role of a particular ASO at an historical moment. The interviews and participant observation data additionally generated a rich seam of information on how different kinds of persons experienced the Centre and each other, and it is this that forms part of the analysis of this book. Various other publications were generated by the research which may be of interest to the reader: the overall evaluation (Bebbington *et al.*, 1992), a qualitative and quantitative appreciation of the volunteer experience (Bebbington and Gatter, 1994), and a critical analysis of the role of psychotherapy at the Centre (Gatter, 1998).

The Centre provided a special kind of environment in which people could explore the meanings of being HIV-positive with others similarly affected. What happened here was probably different from in the community at large, though it may have been repeated in other social care organizations in Britain and perhaps elsewhere where voluntarism is prominent (North America, other European countries). Throughout our research the positive role of the Centre was praised by our interviewees.

In closing this chapter it is worth considering the future. With the advent of new combination therapies, funding is being diverted to treatment rather than care. Organizations such as the Centre are closing down or merging with others. However, unless HIV and AIDS come to be seen as part of a 'normal' range of illness experiences, HIV-positive people will continue to face prejudice, so it is regrettable that places like the Centre will no longer exist to provide a haven in which to re-establish a positive self-image for living with HIV or AIDS. Models of care were developed in the 1980s, often described as possessing 'Rolls Royce' quality, which were innovatory and combined a range of services in a way not previously thought of in relation to other health issues. It seems, unfortunately, that they will become museum pieces rather than vehicles for future development or adoption in new circumstances, experiments sidelined because of considerations of cost and efficiency. This book will, I hope, demonstrate that some of the benefits of places like the Centre can never be reduced to a quantified analysis of costs and benefits. Their wider social significance will not be appreciated from such a perspective.

Notes

1. Throughout the text the organization that was researched is anonymized as the Centre.
2. A total of 58 interviews were conducted with service users, the remaining 12 by Pat Warren.
3. The ONS classifications must be read with caution. Sociologically speaking, some interviewees did not fit easily into these categories, for example someone born into a middle-class family, yet effectively outside the class system after years of injecting drugs use. Similarly, non-British individuals whose class positions in their countries of origin might be very different from here have not been classified.

3

AIDS and the Individual

What image does PWA conjure up? The first time I read the acronym for Person With AIDS I was reminded of POW (Prisoner of War); a coincidence maybe, a simple resemblance, but then, as Susan Sontag has argued, the language of illness is replete with military metaphor (Sontag, 1991, p. 95). PWA is a term invented in America. Like MSM (Men who have Sex with Men) it is a neologism designed in part to neutralize stereotypes. It encourages us to speak of people, not AIDS victims, AIDS queers and so forth. It is a term invented in reaction, but it raises the question of what it means, if anything, to be a person with AIDS. Of course, having AIDS means a lot, but the point for exploration in this chapter is whether PWA has come to denote a meaningful personal identity (complete or partial) and, if so, if the processes of acquiring this identity can be specified. I will be exploring ways in which different kinds of individuals discuss themselves in relation to HIV and AIDS. The following two chapters will contextualize these self-narrations, first in terms of social processes of identity formation: Chapter 4 considers the significance of community. Second, I look at the relations between identity and illness more widely in Chapter 5 by comparing AIDS with other illnesses. This is merely a convenient and conventional way of presenting the argument, and is not intended to suggest that individual and group self-perception are separate phenomena, nor that they should be isolated in comparing AIDS with other experiences of illness. As argued in Chapter 2, identity in late modernity has to be understood as a process that is simultaneously individual and collective.

AIDS as identity signifier

Social scientists, historians, and cultural activists alike have emphasized the symbolic dimensions of AIDS. AIDS is as much a crisis of signification as it is a syndrome related complexly to infection by Human Immunodeficiency Virus, to cite Paula Treichler (1988). The core argument here is that because of the historical association in the metropolitan West between gay men and HIV infection, a particular form of cultural association has been made which draws on a popular construction of sexuality. AIDS is a disease of society since

> As a public health problem, AIDS is a new, unforeseen phenomenon, provoking reactions of panic, revealing social fissures, inequalities and the discrimination and stigmatisation of marginalised groups in society. (Pollak, Paicheler and Pierre, 1992, p. 1)

In Britain, the behaviours of both gay men and injecting drugs users (though for different reasons) have been pathologized. At some level, what both these groups do is conceived as an abuse of nature: gay men subvert the natural sexual use of the body, whereas drugs users poison it. Perhaps most importantly, to these groups are attributed moral as well as physical sickness; indeed these two elements are not discriminated.

These forms of prejudice have a long history predating AIDS, informed by both religious and secular discourses. Homosexuality was a 'sin against nature' in the medieval church (Foucault, 1978). It was also, until the 1970s, regarded as a form of mental illness by the psychiatric profession. By the accident of the epidemiological path it took, AIDS is a frightening contagion, which has been interpreted by conservative moralists as a judgement on perversity and immorality. The response has been most graphic in the United States. Evangelical preachers such as Pat Buchanan and Pat Robertson have explicitly linked AIDS to homosexuality and its supposed threat to the family and American way of life. In the Senate, Jesse Helms has been responsible for preventing the funding of

AIDS organizations via his amendment to stop, in his view, the promotion of homosexuality.[1]

In Britain the activities of the moralist right have been less vituperative, but echo similar sentiments. The evangelical churches have a far smaller following here, yet concern is growing where these churches are establishing themselves in areas with significant lesbian and gay populations. Recently, the attempt by a Brazilian church to purchase the Academy in Brixton (formerly a music venue) drew a strong response in the gay press. Within government the pejorative linking of AIDS to homosexuality was most apparent in the debate leading to the vote in February 1994 on Edwina Currie's Private Member's Bill to lower the gay male age of consent from 21 to 16. Numerous examples of moralizing can be quoted from the proceedings of the debate. Perhaps more insidiously, homosexuality was linked to AIDS in arguments that tried to portray themselves as pragmatic, neutral and scientific. Thus Lady Olga Maitland, sponsor of the Conservative Family Campaign, when asked in an interview for the *Independent* newspaper whether 16-year-old boys were old enough to decide their sexuality:

> In some cases no. You can have boys of 16 who are emotional and very vulnerable. They can be perfectly normal heterosexuals, but if they are going through an awkward time with girls they might mistakenly think they are homosexuals and feel pressurised to yield to homosexual advances which could nudge them into a sexuality which isn't natural to them. That could mean they enter the twilight world of homosexuality and be denied normal family life. Sixteen-year-old girls are much more mature for their age. Also, if a girl has a heterosexual relationship she is not going against her basic nature and is less exposed to AIDS. (Olga Maitland, *Independent*, 20 January 1994)

Many writers have explored what it is about AIDS that makes it a vortex for social and moral concerns. Susan Sontag, for example, argues that AIDS raises our worst fantasies concerning sexuality and death, indeed that AIDS in the West culturally links sexuality to death through illness. Her particular concern has been the way that AIDS and other forms of illness are constructed linguistically, and how this in turn distorts people's perceptions and actions in relation to illness. Popular versions of the biomedical model of disease have been articulated through the military metaphor of invasion:

> The metaphor implements the way particularly dreaded diseases are envisaged as an alien 'other', as enemies are in modern war; and the move from the demonization of the illness to the attribution of fault to the patient is an inevitable one, no matter if patients are thought of as victims. Victims suggest innocence. And innocence, by the inexorable logic that governs all relational terms, suggests guilt. (Sontag, 1978; Penguin edition, 1991, p. 97)

This process occurs only for certain kinds of illness, particularly those for which there is no cure, and which have distressing effects on the body. Crucially, the stigmatization of bearers of illness will happen where responsibility for becoming ill can somehow be made to rest with the ill person, when rightly or wrongly a link is perceived between aspects of a person's lifestyle and proneness to disease. Such putative links can become internalized by the ill: they may believe they are responsible for their illness. Paradoxically, some support organizations for PWAs, at least in the United States, have explicitly worked with a model that blames, or at least makes responsible for having AIDS, the HIV-infected person. So, in *Inventing AIDS*, Cindy Patton is critical of the way that the Twelve Step Programme, originating in Alcoholics Anonymous, has been adopted for PWAs. This model relies on the idea that the person with a 'condition' or 'problem' must first accept responsibility for it, and that the route out of the problem is to give up control to some 'higher power' (Patton, 1990, p. 11). The example suggests that processes of stigmatization are not solely associable with obviously illiberal or censorious forces and institutions.

We, meaning individuals, governments, voluntary organizations, even activists, invest disease with meaning beyond the biological 'facts', and Sontag's aim was to go 'against interpretation', to strip away the layers of culturally loaded meanings that have become attached to certain illnesses. Examining TB and cancer historically, she contrasted the romantic associations of the former with the exclusive repugnance reserved for the latter. What they had in common was that beyond being examples of illness, they were archetypes: cultural symbols for illness, and even death.

Aside from specific behavioural causes of cancer, such as smoking, a more general association has come to be made in this century between emotional repression, a depressive personality, and vulnerability to cancer. Cancer metaphors have led to self-hate and diminution of self among cancer sufferers, since they may come to believe that their own inadequacies have led inexorably to the disease. Cancer is shameful in its meanings, and this can have terrible consequences in terms of patients hiding the disease and refusing to seek treatment.

Sontag later applied this form of analysis to AIDS (Sontag, 1989; Penguin edition, 1991). Unlike cancer, HIV, the generally accepted ultimate causative factor in AIDS, is transmitted between individuals. But this transmission is in blood and sexual fluids, and is culturally linked to ideas of pollution and venereal disease. AIDS links with notions of the clean and unclean, and the boundaries between untamed nature and civilized culture. Such boundaries are important in most human cultures, a theory propounded by the anthropologist Mary Douglas in her seminal *Purity and Danger* (1966).

Transmission of HIV, furthermore, is known to occur only through a small number of quite specific and difficult modes. In the West at least, it is not usually any mystery as to how HIV infection occurred, so there is an easy association to be made between infection and membership of an 'easily' identifiable risk group. The pejorative metaphors of AIDS have been attached to gay men and drugs users (and to some extent sex workers). This raises an interesting question of how HIV and AIDS may be differently experienced by individuals who do not belong to any culturally defined risk group, a theme explored later and in the comparison of AIDS with other chronic illnesses in Chapter 5.

Commentators such as Susan Sontag have carefully explored the cultural backdrop against which someone diagnosed as HIV-positive, or living with AIDS, is positioned. This cultural backdrop, described extensively in cultural studies (e.g. Crimp, 1988) and in cultural productions and commentaries (e.g. Watney, 1987; Gupta and Boffin, 1990), creates a space in which the crisis of becoming the bearer of a powerful stigma may occur, a crisis enveloping the medical trauma of immediate health problems and (generally) reduced life expectancy. Both these crises will enter the self-consciousness of the individual. It is the relationship between them that has not been explored well, due largely to the division in labour between practitioners of cultural studies and social scientists interested in health and illness. In this and the next two chapters I attempt to link the influences of these two crises, by examining the narratives of people living with HIV and AIDS.

First, though, I will introduce some important social science perspectives on the process of stigmatization, which help provide a framework in which to characterize narratives of stigmatizing illness.

Stigmatization, medicalization and resistance

The classic work on stigma in sociology is Erving Goffman's *Stigma: Notes on the Management of Spoiled Identity* (1963). Goffman argues that a stigma is any deeply discrediting attribute of an individual; something which, in cultural and social terms, renders a person less than completely human. Goffman is carefully sociological: stigmatization is not necessarily morally and politically acceptable, but he is interested instead in how particular cultures and societies define for themselves what constitutes human imperfection. And no stigma is universal, since what constitutes a discrediting attribute is socially and relationally defined.

Goffman draws a distinction between the discredited and discreditable individual. The former has a stigmatizing attribute which is immediately apparent, such as a physical deformity. The latter has a less apparent attribute, which to some degree can be hidden. This individual can at least try through 'impression management' to 'pass' as normal. So, a gay man can 'act straight', and someone with partial hearing or sight impairment can use behaviours to mask the attribute (avoiding certain environments, adopting certain body language).

Goffman also defines three different categories of stigmatizing attribute:

1. physical deformities
2. character defects (including homosexuality)
3. race, nation and religion

Depending on whether an individual is discredited or discreditable, these three kinds of attributes relate to three characteristic responses by the stigmatized:

1. The individual may attempt to conceal or correct the stigma.
2. The individual will learn activities not usually thought possible for the person with such a stigma.
3. The individual will reinterpret oppression as the basis of learning and growth through suffering.

Goffman goes beyond the daily management of stigma to consider how the stigmatized deal with their situation over the course of their lives. Individuals become socialized to their stigma through a 'moral career'. This will, with time, usually involve identifying with and forming some kind of social grouping with others similarly stigmatized and sympathetic 'normals' (the *own* and the *wise*). At the social level, a stigmatized individual can also, in Goffman's analysis, be seen to participate in forms of cultural deviance, either as an in-group deviant (someone deviant to a concretely definable group or community), or as a social deviant (someone who in response to stigma rejects the basic institutions of society). Social deviants challenge the legitimacy of, among other things, the family, stereotyped gender role divisions, the age–grade system, segregation by class and race and what constitutes legitimate employment. The category 'social deviant' includes prostitutes, drug addicts, delinquents, criminals, bohemians, gypsies, carnival workers, winos, homosexuals, and the urban unrepentant poor (Goffman, [1963] 1968, p. 170). All of these groups are involved in some kind of collective denial of the social order. Goffman's categorizations were written in the early 1960s, using some terms that today are unacceptably pejorative; his basic framework for analysis, however, remains apposite.

The experience of illness

The works of Sontag and Goffman suggest a theoretical frame within which to consider how social values penetrate self-perception where stigmatizing illness is concerned. A separate and recent body of sociological literature focuses on how clinical aspects of illness reshape people's lives and self-perception in the context of their social networks. This 'experience of illness' literature is expanding to a large number of chronic illnesses. Particular examples are considered in depth in Chapter 5 in posing the question of whether AIDS is a chronic illness like any other. The general approach, as exemplified by Ray Fitzpatrick (1984) is to begin with the onset and diagnosis of an illness, and explore, retrospectively, how this is interpreted by the individual. In comparison with many acute illnesses, onset may be gradual and diagnosis equivocal. The 'ill person', when confronted by a label such as 'multiple sclerosis', may feel a need to develop a personal (and perhaps idiosyncratic) explanatory framework for what was previously a set of vague, intermittent, gradually worsening symptoms. Given the often serious nature of chronic illness in terms of necessary changes to lifestyle and possible reduced life expectancy, the personal aetiology of an illness will often include a rationale for 'why me?'

Central to the experience-of-illness approach is an account of patient coping strategies. Coping is a very important aspect of chronic illness, since biomedical cures may not be available: the sociological emphasis here is on how the *interpretation* of illness events may be as real and significant to the individual as the events themselves. Making sense of what is happening matters as much as the physical experience itself, since chronic illness typically is not a discrete event within what might otherwise be considered a 'normal' life in the same way as acute illness.

Sociologically, coping strategies are analysed in terms of a personal biography related to the progression of illness. An earlier model which typified the chronically ill as going through a four-stage process from denial through gradual acceptance to accommodation with illness (echoing Kubler-Ross's analysis in *On Death and Dying*, 1970) has been challenged by sociologists for whom the empirical evidence is of more complex shifting patterns of what is termed biographical disruption (see Robinson, 1988). This idea of 'biographical disruption' was developed in the early 1980s, and derives from Antony Giddens' term 'critical situation', by which he meant schismatic disturbances to everyday life which help throw into relief the normal and mundane (Giddens, 1979). What Giddens applied originally to situations such as war was transferred to interpreting chronic illness:

> My contention is that illness, and especially chronic illness, is precisely that kind of experience where the structures of everyday life and the forms of knowledge which underpin them are disrupted. (Bury, 1982, p. 169)

Living with pain constantly, and possibly facing an early death, represent a sharp dislocation of the trajectory of a 'normal' life, particularly for the young. As importantly, chronic illness enters and affects the social network of the individual, throwing into relief the nature of personal relationships by exerting new pressures on them. As Bury tellingly noted, chronic illness disrupts the normal, taken-for-granted rules of reciprocity and mutual support (*ibid.*).

Telling stories of illness

Analyses of the cultural meanings of AIDS such as Sontag's suggest a macrosociological space in which a person might make sense of the experience of living with AIDS. Goffman further elaborates the nature of stigma as a social force. The experience-of-illness approach is more microsociological, focusing on the ill person and immediate social networks. In particular, it has analysed relations between medical professionals and the ill person, and the ways in which medical knowledge becomes incorporated in lay interpretations of illness. All of these approaches may be useful in guiding the analysis of individuals' experiences of HIV and AIDS.

The experiences I will relate here and analyse are drawn from interviews with 46 people, varying from those HIV-positive but asymptomatic to some in advanced stages of illness.[2] The interviews formed part of the evaluation of the Centre, as outlined in Chapter 2. Interviews were semi-structured, and geared to developing a detailed picture of experiences of HIV-related services across statutory and voluntary sectors. They began, however, by inviting the respondents to explore, in a discursive way, how HIV had affected their lives; to tell their story. That the interviews were part of a service evaluation was made explicit by me, so it is likely that this context will have shaped the emphases placed by individuals on particular experiences. It was clear at some points that my role as researcher was perceived as a possible conduit for complaints. Nevertheless, the interview structure meant that there was considerable space for narration, and respondents were only later guided to focus specifically on HIV service experiences and requirements.

The interviews provided accounts of diverse persons, experiences and contexts. Their detail ranges from daily medication routines to profound changes in self-consciousness and sense of purpose in life. For the purposes of this chapter I will discuss those emergent themes that relate in some sense to self-identity. The illustrative quotations that follow are not in any sense statistically representative, but rather are chosen as particular exemplars of themes prominent in a number of accounts. Some brief biographical details are given with each quotation where these will aid the reader contextually, but to preserve confidentiality they are kept to a minimum. For the same reason I have also modified some trivial details. Quotations from interviews are used again in Chapter 4 to pursue aspects of group identity, with the same methodological intent and discretions.

Statements made by interviewees are taken at face value. I have not attempted to search for latent meanings (as a psychological approach might require), nor to apply any form of discourse analysis to the texts of transcribed interviews. In relation to the discussion that follows, the themes of diagnosis, biographical disruption and so forth are examined in the low-level theoretical sense in which they are presented in the 'experience of illness' literature. For the interested reader, there is a growing body of work that aims at a more metatheoretical treatment; in particular, the application of a Foucauldian concept of discourse to the medicalization of people living with chronic illnesses, and the counter-discourses (resistance) that they develop in relation to biomedicine. An application of such theory in the context of HIV and AIDS is well developed in the work of Brian Heaphy (see Heaphy, 1996, 1998). For further examples of interviews with individuals living with HIV/AIDS in the 'experience of literature' frame, but in the context of the United States, see Weitz (1991) and Adam and Sears (1996).

The event of a positive HIV diagnosis is a reasonable starting point: in almost all interviews, respondents chose this as the opening for their narratives.

Diagnosis

Retrospectively, HIV diagnosis was described, with few exceptions, as a shock, a schism, though not always a nightmare. The factors affecting the nature of the experience were a mixture of personal circumstance and historical trajectory.

There has undoubtedly been a large improvement in standard and consistency of HIV testing and counselling services in Britain since antibody tests first became available in the mid-1980s. The longest diagnosed interviewees had, with the exception of those attending the leading treatment centres in central London, experienced a lack of support surrounding diagnosis, which influenced their ability to cope subsequently. Little pre- or post-test counselling was offered, doctors revealed diagnoses insensitively, individuals saw 'HIV Positive' written about them on records that were not fully confidential. A bad experience of the testing procedure and bureaucracy was seen, after the event, as foundational for life afterwards. In a few cases, such experiences formed the focus for continuing rage at the medical profession, even years afterwards.

> I went to ... hospital at the end of ... with an ear infection. I was in for 4 to 5 days. The place was filthy. I was tested for HIV without my knowledge and then just given the result. I was very upset. My girlfriend found out what had happened by accident. She saw my medical notes, which had been left lying there, saying 'Prepare Mr ... for a diagnosis.' We were both completely shocked.
>
> I wanted to complain about the way I was treated at the hospital. It seems too late now. It makes me so angry. My sexual life has been ruined. My girlfriend won't have sex with me anymore. (Heterosexual man)

Such accounts may embellish what actually happened, and even be interpreted by AIDS professionals as misplaced anger due to the psychological stresses of living with HIV. They also do not draw solely on personal experience. The respondent quoted was a heterosexual man from another European country who did not use HIV-related services, partly because of his dislike of gay men and sense that service centres were gay dominated. His experience of HIV was largely confined to himself and his partner. Yet there were others whose experiences of and feelings about diagnosis were mediated through discussion with other HIV-positive people; they had historicized their experiences socially, either through their existing social networks or through use of HIV-related services. This social experience I will return to, as it was a marked feature of the changing sense of self in interviews.

Whatever the nature of the diagnosis experience, and irrespective of the factuality of the account rendered at interview, diagnosis tended to mark the first fixed point on a map of personal experience of HIV. It was least marked among gay men whose lives had already been affected through the diagnoses and illness of friends, lovers and partners.

> It was kind of a relief in a strange way. I had several friends who were HIV-positive. When I told them they said 'join the club'. In a way I'd have been surprised if I wasn't positive.

Even for these individuals, though, diagnosis represented some sense of separation as well as membership. Fear of HIV was and remains common in parts of the gay community (as elsewhere) and I was given several accounts of malicious disclosure of HIV status in gay social venues, which led to shunning and exclusion of the positive individual.

People who tested positive after the diagnosis of a partner were not only gay men. Among those interviewed were injecting drugs users (heterosexual) and partners of sub-Saharan Africans. What set them apart from gay men was the sense in which their experience of HIV was more socially isolated, as in the case quoted above. Some did not belong to social networks in which being HIV-positive was reckoned possible, let alone probable or acceptable. Their coping mechanisms, beyond partners and immediate family, were very much dependent on voluntary sector HIV organizations.

For others whose lives had not been directly touched by HIV prior to their own diagnosis, a number of patterns were discernible in the circumstances of diagnosis. The first of these was taking the test as a means of identifying the cause of otherwise unexplained (and persistent) ill health. The receipt of a positive diagnosis in this situation had a number of cross-cutting effects. Negatively, the news contained the information of likely further illness and reduced life expectancy. Positively, a label, an identity, had been attached to something that previously had been distressing in part precisely because it had been mysterious:

> There was the most bizarre thing, the most immense relief, that finally I realized that the stress I'd been under for all these years had been building and building. Now I knew the worst. Not alone was I HIV, but I was sort of AIDS. So I mean it can't get worse than that. (Gay man, in his forties, who suspected he might have been infected in the USA in the early 1980s)

Such experiences are similar to many reported in the literature of experience of illness and sociology of chronic illness. A further parallel lies in the felt need to trace back from the moment of diagnosis to an assumed point of infection. Since this group of interviewees were ill at the time of diagnosis, they recognized that they may have been HIV-positive for some years previously. Nearly all offered some kind of account of how and when they may actually have been infected. Similar narratives are recorded, for example, from people living with multiple sclerosis. What perhaps differentiates HIV and AIDS from other illnesses in this respect is the idea of a latent period which may last in excess of a decade,[3] during which there is no revelation of illness or difference. The accounts from my interviewees were not just about the onset of mysterious illness: they were an attempt to mark an event in time which could only be known about (or guessed at) retrospectively.

> HIV first affected me right back in 1982, when *Horizon* did the first programme that was ever done on AIDS on television. I seem to be the only person who ever saw it. And on it you saw, I mean, I'm haunted to this day by this young black guy in Atlanta going for tests with an awful ongoing stomach problem and diarrhoea. It said later he has since died. And there was all the things they knew about, you know, multiple sexual partners, and the difficult areas, San Francisco, New York, Los Angeles. And I had been there, and they thought at the time there was a sort of incubation period of one to two years. I had been in Los Angeles, San Francisco, New York for four months in 1980. Well, I was absolutely terrified, because I'd gone to the bath houses and everything there. I thought there was no way I can have escaped. (As above)

This pattern supports the view that the events both of infection and diagnosis mark an important critical event in the narrative of the self, even though the former may be an invention or rationalization.

A third group of interviewees discovered they were HIV-positive through what might be described as contingent circumstances: neither through illness nor because of the positive status of a sexual or injecting drugs-using partner. These included the 'worried well': those who had been tested because they had practised unsafe sex or were uncertain of the risks attaching to their sexual practices. Some gay men, embarking on what they expected to be a monogamous relationship, decided to be tested as a couple so that, supposing they both tested negative, they might have the option of practising unprotected anal sex. There were a few others who decided to test because they had been encouraged to do so within their social networks, because AIDS figured in their concerns as the worried well. For them, the event of a positive diagnosis came as a complete surprise. Discovery of HIV-positive status was more shocking to them than for others:

> It was a bit of a joke actually at the time 'cause friends of mine, there was four of us, and two of them had previously been going out together, one came down ill and it was, 'cause we didn't know very much about HIV or AIDS. We all thought he might have AIDS, so it's like well we all should go along as support, help him through it and if he is diagnosed with HIV, then we should help 'cause we're friends, we'll stick together. We were encouraged to go along. I was a bit hesitant at first, but then I thought well why not, just to shut him up. I passed the STD test, and they said to me do you want to go on and have the HIV test? And I was like yes, why not. Then when I found out it was a shock, but it was a secret I kept to myself, for about two years.

Later:

> And with me, I just live life for each day. I always make sure not to relate what I'm feeling to what I've got and that's important for everybody to believe in. (Gay man in his mid-twenties)

Those interviewees who had recently been diagnosed under these conditions would tend to say that they were not letting HIV interfere with their lives; that there was no need to accept that anything had changed. Those interviewed at a later time tended to regard the period shortly after diagnosis as one of denial, since diagnosis had come as such a shock.

Life projects disrupted

In their narratives, my interviewees often explicitly followed an account of HIV diagnosis with how this disrupted their sense of future selfhood – a classic aspect of biographical disruption. A general feeling of intimation of untimely mortality took root in a number of related areas which might be termed projects of life.

> Sometimes I see an old friend for a drink, and I try to act like normal and it's very difficult sometimes when people start talking about long-term things that they are going to do and they talk about this or other problems which really, when you're living with a life or death situation, not just you personally but people you know, it becomes all rather trite, you know, it's difficult to be enthusiastic about what they see as problems. On another level, a lot of it has to do with finances. My biggest problem since being diagnosed and not being at work: it's affected my social life more than anything. (Heterosexual man)

This kind of sense of loss was common across categories of interviewees; particular life projects tended to differentiate them. So, for example, heterosexuals who had perceived their lives in terms of raising a (conventional) family felt confronted by the likelihood of no longer being able to have children because of the risk of vertical transmission of HIV from mother to child where both partners were positive, or where infection of a previously HIV-negative woman might result from trying to become pregnant. For those who had not yet become parents, there was a sense of having been robbed of something important:

> The main thing for me is that we wanted to have children, and now we can't. I can't be a father. That is a terrible thing. (Heterosexual man)

For those who already had children the problems emphasized were of not being able to fulfil the parental role for their children until those children reached adulthood and independence, and of reversing roles so that, in times of illness, they might find themselves dependent on their children. This theme was made even more poignant in the case of a couple who had also been injecting drugs users:

> When they found out about us, automatically they decide everything for themselves without consulting us or anything [to adopt granddaughter]. They say, oh you know it's no good for B to be

going here and there, if she gets ill. You are waiting for housing and this and that. She should stay with us. The more time goes on the more it's like we've lost our daughter and sometimes we'll be talking about it and we think should we ask for her back, and what sort of problems would happen if we did? What if I get ill or he gets ill and we also have to keep going to hospital and things?

We don't even know if she's positive. I presume she's not positive because she hasn't been ill. I'm worried then that if both of us die, she won't really remember us very well. I can leave her a tape, you know, letters and things that might put some of my perceptions, but it's not the same thing as if I had her here. I wouldn't want her to see me dying, but at least she would remember Mum and Dad in a better way and not ask so many questions when she grows up. (Mother discussing her daughter)

HIV status raised wider problems of loss connected with sexuality. All sexually active respondents reported fears of the prospect of infecting someone else, at least in the period after diagnosis. Some had partners who left them after their diagnoses, either through fears of transmission, or of not being able to cope with the emotional demands of living with someone whose health might gradually deteriorate. For a few, there was an abiding sense of no longer being a sexual being; that the risks, however small, meant involuntary celibacy, or at the least that it would be difficult to find sexual partners while being honest about HIV status. In spite of the arguments for and against disclosure of status in casual sexual relationships, nearly all the respondents in the study felt a strong need to disclose to sexual partners, especially where there was any perceived risk involved in sexual activities. These findings resemble research conducted by Sigma Research, using focus groups, into the sexual health needs of HIV-positive gay and bisexual men (Keogh *et al.*, 1995, pp. 18–19).

With time, this sense of desexualization often wore off so that sexual careers were begun again in the context of safer sexual practices, or unprotected sex by agreement between HIV-positive partners. Gay men were, interestingly, both the most and least affected respondents in terms of loss of sexual self. For those who had withdrawn sexually, the loss was especially acute: most of the gay men in the study were active in the inner urban gay scene in London, and participated in highly sexualized social and cultural networks. To be no longer sexual was to be alienated in two senses. Within the Centre gay men tended to congregate and socialize in the drop-in area, where sexuality and sexual activity formed a staple of daily conversation. So to be non-sexual created problems for general social interaction as well as sense of sexual self. On the other hand, it was among gay men that there was, generally speaking, the highest level of knowledge about HIV prevention, and a sense of HIV as an accepted part of life, something familiar. Thus, some gay men in the study had HIV-negative partners for whom HIV was not a problem; others had found positive partners through their networks on the scene.

These observations on gay men suggest that loss of sexual self can be seen as residing within a wider category of loss of social self. Here, Goffman's ideas about stigma become relevant. Although in the wider community some gay respondents experienced prejudice in which being gay was seen as equivalent to having AIDS (several horror stories were told regarding life on inner London housing estates), within personal social and sexual networks (the immediate gay community) there was relatively little stigma. It was among other categories of respondent, such as refugee Africans, that social withdrawal associated with stigma was reported.

I have used the term 'withdrawal' here deliberately, since in Goffman's terms what respondents described was being discreditable, rather than discredited – that they were acting on felt rather than enacted stigma. Some of the East African women interviewed had withdrawn from contact with other members of their community in London for fear of being outcast should their status become known to others. In their home countries being HIV-positive was associated with being a bad and immoral person, such as a sex worker. For others: ex-IDUs and non-community-attached gay and bisexual men, the rationales for withdrawal were rather different. In and of itself, unpredictable health (general fatigue and acute episodes) imposed restrictions on social activity, but further self-imposed restriction came through fear that a progressive deterioration in health and refusal of social engagements would draw suspicion and eventual revelation of HIV status. Fear of this eventuality led to an early severing of social ties, perhaps to be replaced with new connections through HIV-related organizations.

This form of withdrawal took a particular form amongst ex-IDUs, though here it was the drug-taking habit that assumed greater significance than HIV status. Maintaining the status *ex-user* in relation to drugs depended on staying away from previous social circles of users, and this pattern was reinforced by the knowledge that further drugs use when HIV-positive would contribute to a hastened decline in health.

> It is one of the most difficult problems for people who have been taking drugs on a regular basis when they stop, because it really is a vacuum. All your old friends – if you continue to meet them but want to stay off drugs it's really tough. It means stopping seeing a lot of people, people you might like a lot. Plus, if they find out you're positive, and knowing you were involved in the same circle, they might freak out. (Heterosexual ex-drugs-user)

A particularly acute sense of personal and social loss was experienced by those whose friends and partners had died with AIDS. Repeatedly, gay respondents referred to a form of 'grief fatigue' and a collective sense of loss of community which amounted to a diminished self. Non-gay respondents were less likely to be involved in networks affected by HIV, except where they had subsequently become involved with HIV organizations.

> When my grandmother died I never cried at all, and I went to the funeral. Never shed a tear. I put it down to seeing so much death anyway, especially working on acute medical wards, and losing so many of my close friends through AIDS. I suppose I've come to accept death, it's inevitable. But then, when R died you've never seen anyone cry as much as I did. R was more or less the first person I met when I came to London. We had a little fling together, which just didn't work, like chalk and cheese. But we've remained friends ever since. And then to suddenly lose him was just a big shock. I just got this telephone call to say he'd died. I cried, but it wasn't until I got into the church, and heard the music he'd picked for his funeral, well, that was it, I just burst into tears walking through the door and sobbed my heart out right through the whole of his funeral. (Gay man in his forties)

Loss of a long-term partner affected sense of self in a distinctive way, though one that could be associated with such loss in any circumstance, regardless of the presence of HIV.

I didn't realize how dependent I was on my partner. I thought in fact that, although we were very very close, that we were two distinct people, which we were in a way. And it wasn't until after my partner died that I realized how interrelated in everything we were, and that was then much around relationships as well. I mean, I've had a lot of support, but I've often found it difficult to accept. My partner and I had been together such a long time (29 years), when we were with others we complemented one another. We knew when to go and what signals to make when we were with people. We were mutually supportive most of the time. Yes, it's a realization that came very strongly to me after. I didn't realize how strongly I interdepended.

Work was one further significant area in which respondents described loss of self. Once illness entered the picture, withdrawal from work could be a choice, or an inevitability. The rationale for such withdrawal, and what it meant to someone, varied considerably with their circumstances: individual illness interacted with work context. In some instances stopping work was forced by physical collapse and subsequent medical advice. More often the process of withdrawal was less dramatic and involved elements of choice by the individual.

Again, felt stigma played a role. Frequent illness and sick leave was perceived as possibly leading to suspicion among work colleagues about the underlying cause. This could precipitate a decision to resign as much as any physical debilitation, though usually the decision was informed also by medical advice that the avoidance of work-related stress should help to prolong good health.

It was unusual for an interviewee to have taken lightly the decision to stop work. The economic consequences were justifiably feared, especially among professional and managerial people for whom the drop in income and change in lifestyle implied by life on state benefits was enormous. Though they might have good private or occupational pensions, few were of an age where they would yet benefit much from these, and many insurance policies would not pay out for retirement forced through illness where HIV might be identified as the cause.

I've got a large mortgage and that's the only thing that fucks me off in life. Now if I got rid of that tomorrow, I mean I could tell them at work and retire. I want to retire on medical grounds, but I'm not unwell and don't want to pretend to be. If I didn't go to work I think I might become a voluntary worker, helping people, be a buddy or something like that. But it's having the mortgage fucks me up. I'd still like to be independent of the state. I'd like to have my lump sum and my pension from the office. But if I retired I wouldn't have enough to pay off the mortgage. I suppose I would have, with the right policies and scraping every penny, but I'd have nothing to live on except whatever state benefit there is. (Gay man in his forties in a professional occupation)

Income was directly related to capacity to participate in valued social activities, and fear of poverty kept some people in work beyond a point at which doctors had advised retirement. Further down the income scale fears persisted, but, for those on low incomes who were AIDS diagnosed, it was possible that they would receive more in enhanced benefits than they were previously paid in wages.

Beyond income itself, work was strongly tied to feelings of self-worth. In different ways, respondents from a range of socio-economic categories expressed the need to work as a sign of full adult citizenship. To work was to be independent and a contributor to society. There was a fear that dependence on the state amounted to a loss of agency, a personal failing. This kind of concern was voiced across differences of class.

Work. I think it's important to everybody. You know £35 a week on the unemployed is, you know, no good. And I've always worked. This is the first time I've ever not worked. And that's because I have Kaposi's on my legs and I get tired and stuff now. But I just carried on working. I think that's the best thing for everybody. There's a lot to say you know when they chuck people out of their jobs. I've always felt for them because it's quite a dramatic thing in someone's life. Then to feel that you've got no references or stuff like that. (Working-class gay man, formerly working in catering industry)

I've never been dependent on anyone. I know it's a snobbish thing to say, but I look at some of the people who come to the Centre. They live on benefits, they've never done anything with their lives.

I don't want to be like that. (Middle-class, professional gay man in his thirties)

Among the professionals, there was also the sense of work as a predominant expression of self, that to stop work was not only to enter a void of unfilled time, but to have no life project with which to fill this void. It was, however, this group for whom work context provided the greatest protections, especially where work was in health services, local authorities, or voluntary organizations. Two managers in such settings had been able to negotiate phased withdrawal from work, beginning with working from home, in a setting where they were able to be open about HIV status (their employers had equal opportunities policies which encompassed HIV).

A: Until January it was full-time. But travelling around the country a lot. Now I'm negotiating to go back part-time, doing some work from home, two days a week. Just to sort of slowly get back into it.
Q: Is it difficult to do that?
A: No. It's a care-giving charity and they have a very positive attitude. (Manager in a caring charity)

Both these respondents were in quite high positions within their organizations, and their experiences around work and retirement were the most positive reported, in terms both of personal and financial consequences. An analysis of the personal experience of HIV in relation to work must therefore include consideration of the wider institutional context in which work takes place. In this respect, public sector employers in Britain have in general taken a more supportive stance than the private sector, though even here the values and attitudes of individual employers influence the outcomes.

All the interviewees who had been working at the time of diagnosis were men, except for two professional women who were asymptomatic at the time of interview and continuing in work. Others interviewed were unemployed, or had a history of casual work and economic marginality. In general, switching to living on health-related benefits did not figure as a major schism to them, though some casual workers wished, if health allowed, to work now and again to boost income. For a few, whose lifestyles were marginal through drugs use, mental health problems and other reasons, having access to health benefits represented, if anything, a new-found security. They had not seen themselves previously as part of a culture of work.

> The biggest change really is, I feel in some ways that HIV in a way has been the best thing that's ever happened to me. Because I always had problems with being able to cope with work. I couldn't handle it and I could never fit in to this world as society expected it. And HIV came along, and now of course I don't have to come up with excuses for not working. I suppose now I feel more settled, and I suppose I've got more idea of where I'm going. (Gay man in his thirties)

Life projects regained

So far I have referred to the ways in which interviewees described what might be labelled diminished selves. These were common features of a variable period after diagnosis. Some more isolated people continued to reinforce their isolation through progressive social withdrawal. Fear of disclosure and loss could become a self-fulfilling prophecy. For many others, though, a point was reached at which some kind of reorganization around life priorities began to emerge; life projects were regained, albeit rather different ones than before diagnosis. This self-reconstruction was realized through several channels, connecting an inner sense of self with a redeveloped social identity. Significantly, these channels were linked in that life projects often grew out of initial dialogues with others. I will consider the development of individual projects and then describe the wider social context they are mediated through in Chapter 4. In all these processes a common theme is the accommodation to 'living with HIV'.

Respondents who narrated regained life projects spoke of themselves as individuals, and as members of a more abstract group, as being 'HIV positive', 'living with HIV', or even just 'HIV' (used adjectivally). They spoke with some degree of identification with HIV. It is likely that this group would be identified by a psychologist as having moved beyond a period of denial, towards adjustment and acceptance, a commonly identified feature of diagnosis and aftermath with potentially life-threatening chronic illnesses. Such individual psychological processes are of great significance to coping strategies, but my chosen focus is identity formation and transformation, rather than psychological equilibrium. Thus, though the following discussion is framed in terms of regaining and reconstituting, there is no intention of implying any direct correlation with psychological or physical well-being.

'Owning' HIV

In Goffman's terms, my interviewees came to see themselves as belonging with others through HIV status, to see these others as their 'own'. But ownership of HIV also took the form of possession and purpose for a sub-group of them. They spoke of something approximating a rite of passage. Turning the stigma, distress, isolation and negativity of being HIV positive on its head, they instead made HIV a vocation, working for others in similar situations, or even to change societal attitudes. Philip Kayal, describing Gay Men's Health Crisis (GMHC) in New York, reported similar motivations for volunteering in an AIDS organization, among both HIV-positive and HIV-negative volunteers (Kayal, 1993).

Working in some capacity for an HIV/AIDS organization was the commonest form this ownership took. Many of the volunteers at the Centre were themselves HIV-positive; others worked as buddies for the Terrence Higgins Trust, or volunteered in other organizations, such as Body Positive.

> The progression from that was our association with a local group around HIV, and being buddies to other people, and helping to develop that voluntary group, and so getting to know a lot of people with HIV, and working around that. There's now a conscious effort to say I don't want to go back to [paid] work. I live on a small pension and my benefits. Most of the past five years [after losing partner to AIDS] has been spent either working as a volunteer or in the development of an HIV/AIDS voluntary organization. (Gay man on a growing association with HIV work)

In a few cases this commitment to HIV led to paid employment in the sector, often for voluntary organizations, but also in health and local authority care settings.

I progressed from voluntary work to being HIV co-ordinator for a health authority. But that nearly killed me, what with all the political infighting. (Gay man)

No, it's got better [of work life]. It's wonderful. HIV has been really good for me in one sense, because it's allowed me to change direction and get out of a rut. (Gay man working in nursing)

In this second case the person had been motivated by his positive HIV status to go on courses relating to HIV/AIDS care, and found it easier to be critical of and stand up to his superiors if he felt they were wrong. His professional self-esteem had increased (though his managers may have perceived the change less positively!).

Owning HIV took other creative forms. Writing about HIV to raise public consciousness, or joining treatment activist groups, such as ACT UP or Positively Healthy, was a response to perceived governmental inactivity; a means of fighting, rather than suffering stigma. In one notable case an individual had founded a theatre company to represent and dramatize experiences of AIDS.

Most of my energy is raising awareness, and I am using the theatre, and writing, in order to try and do something about changing people's attitudes. Part of the ethos of the theatre company, which I set up, is to promote positive images about living with AIDS, but also to raise awareness amongst the general population.

A well-known tabloid newspaper heard the story and wanted to run it with some photographs:

They took some pictures of me as ... and they said, well, you know, in order to do the before and after, we need someone who looks sick. He's an actor. Can you ask him whether he'll make up to look sick. I said tell them to shove it up their arse. (Heterosexual man)

These activities helped regain a sense of control and purpose in life. The most combative among my interviewees turned this critical armoury on the medical profession as well as the government and tabloid press.

Medical knowledge of HIV and its activity in the body is far from complete; and there is in any case no cure. The expert status of medical knowledge was often called into question, with comments such as 'I know much more than the doctors do about what it means to live with HIV'. There was a wish not to be used as a guinea-pig in the pursuit of improved medical knowledge – to be an agent, rather than a patient. The individual quoted above had the following to say, concerning a muscle biopsy and shared care arrangements:

> His [the doctor's] senior registrar walked in and said, 'Oh, P, I was down in London last week, and I was talking to J, and she said oh, we're arranging a muscle biopsy for P.' I turned round to my doctor and said 'You see what I mean?' They just take all control away from you, and say, well, he needs a muscle biopsy, get him booked in. Well, you can fuck off, you do to me what I want you to do to me. And if I don't want you to do anything, I don't even want you talking about it.[4]

A space for lay persons to challenge the authority of doctors is a feature in other chronic illnesses with imperfect treatments and indeterminate prognoses, a subject for detailed discussion in Chapter 5. What is perhaps distinctive about AIDS has been the rapid development and instability of clinical knowledge, and the way it has been communicated both to the medical profession and people living with AIDS.

> Even at a clinical level changes in knowledge about AIDS and how to treat it were so rapid that patients were sometimes as well informed as their doctors and the old 'doctor knows best' approach proved difficult to sustain. (Bennett and Ferlie, 1994, p. 149)

Unusually, new clinical findings often were reported in the popular press before they appeared in medical journals, encouraging the sort of assertive approach to knowing about AIDS and how to deal with doctors exhibited by my interviewee.

A counterpoint to this challenging of medical authority in our study was a growth in interest in complementary therapies. Some respondents used these just because they were available through voluntary organizations, might be worth trying and could do no harm, that is they were used opportunistically. For a few, however, complementary therapy came to represent an expression of faith, a new framework within which to reconstitute and understand the body in its struggle against illness.

Refiguring the body

In the absence of cures for HIV, the importance of bolstering the immune system is recognized by allopathic and complementary medicine alike. Changes in lifestyle such as reducing or ceasing to use alcohol and tobacco, getting sufficient sleep and exercise, eating a carefully balanced diet, are common elements in health advice on living with HIV. A few respondents went much further in lifestyle changes, out of a crisis in faith in the capabilities of biomedicine. Their focus became what might better be described as alternative, rather than complementary therapies. An intense interest developed in non-Western forms, such as Chinese and Ayurvedic medicine, and other kinds of herbalism, together with physical therapies such as reflexology, shiatsu and acupuncture.

> Q: How do you find yourself spending your time now?
> A: Well, I do a lot of reading. Getting into health things again with the support group, I was interested in alternative, holistic ideas. But I didn't know anything about them. And gradually, through the support group, I got to know more about them, and I'm getting right into dowsing now. And I do an awful lot of reading on that. And psychology and different stuff. And programmes about alternative treatments on the telly.
> Q: Do you think alternative therapies have helped you?
> A: Yes, they've done more good than anything else without a doubt. I mean, there's not a lot you can do with HIV except what they call constitutional strengthening to support the immune system. (Gay man in his thirties)

This interest took the form of reading widely, and experiencing the therapies where available. It could also be manifested in joining one of the 'fringe' groups, which promoted such therapies explicitly as a counter-discourse to conventional biomedicine, such that the personal also became political. These groups included the heterodox organization Positively Healthy, which provided alternative treatments and campaigned against the pharmaceutical industry, and produced a newsletter promulgating its philosophy, *Quack Quack Quack*. Also controversial was the *Continuum* newsletter which supported alternative therapies, but also situated itself within 'AIDS Dissidence' since it refused the connection between HIV infection and AIDS.[5]

The embracing of alternative systems of medicine was, when clearly articulated as a strategy running counter to conventional medicine, a way to regain control of the body in the face of the apparent failure of conventional therapies, and against becoming a medicalized 'victim'. The attraction of the philosophies of alternative systems of medicine lay in ideas of balance between the individual and the environment; a holism that has become an attraction of alternative systems of thought in late modernity generally. Respondents stressed also how the nature of interaction with the therapist was very different from a conventional consultation; it involved an opportunity to explore a personal narrative, which helped make sense of the experience of living with HIV, as well as reflecting a more respectful and attentive attitude on the part of the therapist than was sometimes experienced in hospital and clinic settings.

> The therapies have definitely helped . . . with the general fatigue I was getting. I was very very tired all the time. They've helped me with having a better attitude to things. And I feel much calmer. I really feel I'm getting back to what's really me. And I feel more secure in me, not as my child's mother, not as my husband's wife, but in me.
>
> I find that the holistic practitioners are counsellors as well. They listen to you. They spend a lot of time talking. The homoeopath gives me strategies. He's been much more positive than the hospital doctors.

This woman, a mother who had lost her partner, was contrasting her positive experience of alternative therapies and practitioners with an unpleasant perinatal episode in which she had been quarantined and shunned (which is quoted from in Chapter 5).

The point to be stressed here is that although seeking alternative/complementary therapies could be merely opportunistic, or a pursuit of something that conventional medicine had failed to provide, it could equally be a project for salvaging a sense of self, after years of tests, clinic visits, operations, participation in drugs trials and so forth. As one respondent put it, 'the last thing I want is to have the professional title "ill person" '. It is unsurprising that the few respondents who could be thus classified nearly all had AIDS-defining diagnoses and had experienced years of allopathic monitoring and treatment. It was among these people also that one other distinctive form of self-renewal was found.

These examples have to be contrasted with a few respondents who had a decidedly sceptical view of alternative and complementary therapies.

> I don't think you need to dress it up, you know, and wear kimonos and have burning incense. Fine if that's what people want, but it's certainly not for me and I don't ... I'm just so sceptical about things like crystal therapy. (Gay man)

The speaker here was contrasting scepticism about therapies with no obvious physical effects with others such as massage and acupuncture where he felt the evidence in their favour was good. He also emphasized scepticism about the promoters of therapies as much as the therapies themselves. He was concerned that quacks might be promoting unproven therapies to vulnerable people, making them feel that they were not caring for themselves properly if they didn't use such therapies.

> unless you're having aromatherapy, crystal therapy, reflexology, shiatsu or whatever, then you're not doing well. You're not looking after yourself.

This interviewee articulated most strongly a distrust of alternative medicine. He was in a minority, and as a worker within allopathic medicine, might be expected to incline to these views. The few other interviewees who thought little of alternative and complementary therapies generally did so on the grounds that they had tried them and experienced no obvious benefits.

Other studies by social scientists help in delineating the relationship between AIDS and complementary medicine. Ursula Sharma's ethnography of complementary practitioners and patients in the Stoke-on-Trent area of England considers a wide range of clients and illnesses, though none of them were seeking therapy for AIDS-related diseases. She found that in nearly all cases her interviewees first sought complementary therapies because of some intractable medical problem that did not respond to conventional therapy (Sharma, 1992, p. 36). Beyond initial contact with therapists, she identified a number of patterns of usage, for example eclectic use of a variety of therapies, or regular use of one therapy for one problem (*ibid.*, p. 55). As in the present study, she also reported a positive evaluation of relationships with complementary therapists, explicitly contrasted with experiences of conventional therapists:

> To the extent that the practitioner's discourse replaces orthodox explanations with meanings and interpretations which are more satisfactory to the patient, and provides evidence consistent with those meanings, then they may be said to 'work', although not in any clinical sense. (*ibid.*, p. 71)

Her emphasis here is on perceptions of the therapy as shaped by relations with the therapist. The theme of refiguring the body and gaining a sense of control *contra* orthodox practice did not feature as strongly in her study as in ours. The difference, I would argue, lies in the special meanings and significance of AIDS.

Sharma's interviewees, like mine, sought out complementary therapies for chronic, or at least intractable problems (opportunistic infections in AIDS, though technically acute, take on a chronic character because of damage to the immune system). Typically the complaints of Sharma's 'patients' were, however, not life-threatening, whereas AIDS definitely was at the time of our study. This may explain why Sharma found that complementary therapy use was largely pragmatic and opportunistic and not, taking issue with a study by Coward (Coward, 1989, p. 197), related to any novel belief system about the body and health. Only a few interviewees, who could be defined as belonging to a middle-class intelligentsia, propounded such beliefs in Sharma's study (Sharma, 1992, p. 87). In contrast we found a number of people living with HIV or AIDS who had embraced complementary therapy with an enthusiasm bordering on the religious. There was no obvious connection between adopting such beliefs and education, class or upbringing. Tentatively, I suggest that this more elaborated relationship between some people living with HIV and AIDS and the use of complementary therapies (and approval of complementary practitioners), going beyond pragmatic concern with the perceived efficacy of therapies, reflects the fact that AIDS was perceived at the time of our study as being almost inevitably fatal (though with an ill-defined prognosis) and highly stigmatizing. Under such circumstances, belief in an alternative frame for understanding AIDS, and the imagination of a more positive outcome in light of this frame, clearly will be attractive to someone who can make such a 'leap of faith' against a dominant biomedical definition of the problem. The clearest parallels are with other life-threatening and potentially stigmatizing illnesses, such as the turn to complementary or unorthodox therapies in the face of apparently untreatable cancers. The status of alternative treatment centres for cancer, such as the Bristol Cancer Help Centre (see also Chapter 5), remains controversial, and conventional practitioners have argued via examples of public figures or celebrities, such as Steve McQueen, that lives were lost (or lost unnecessarily early) because of a refusal of conventional treatment.

As with cancer, so with AIDS: decisions about treatment exist in a highly politicized context. The problem of defining what AIDS is, and what to do about it, exists for the individual HIV-positive person, but, as we have already seen, is mediated by connections with others. The public dimension of this experience is the theme of the next chapter, but the formation of 'new social worlds' is an important feature of the regaining of self for individuals living with HIV/AIDS. Before discussing this phenomenon there is one further area of experience to note: spirituality and religious belief (as conventionally defined) and their effects on self-perception in relation to HIV/AIDS.

Spirituality

A minority of our interviewees had been practising Christians or adherents of other religions prior to diagnosis. In later stages of illness, in parallel with a turning to alternative therapies, this particular group tended to focus on and redevelop a sense of spirituality in their lives. This was at a point beyond which medicine could offer only a palliative, and dying had become a daily, rather than remote concern. Spirituality was explicitly discussed as a means of coming to terms with death, through imagining a transcendence of the end of bodily existence.

> My friends and family all know it's a possibility that my life might be shorter than I'd prefer it to be, and it's all right because we're Christians. My faith's a very important part of my life. I don't

know how people who are faced with what I'm facing manage to find the strength without faith. I'm not afraid of dying anymore. (Gay man in his fifties)

And in a slightly different key:

Q: Has your faith supported you, I mean in terms of facing illness, thinking about dying?
A: Oh, very much so. Because I'm firmly convinced that when God wants me I will go, no matter what people do. And that this is not the end of everything, it's the beginning of the next part of my existence, if you like. It's difficult to put into words. But I mean, I'll give you an example. With all this problem with the mortgage, I got into bed one night and looked at a picture that I've got of Our Lady, and said 'I think I've had enough, can't take any more of this.' Two days later Welfare Rights got in touch with pay. Now, if that wasn't a prayer answered, I don't know what is. (Roman Catholic gay man in his forties)

Religious or quasi-religious beliefs were more widely raised in interviews where the subject of death arose, including previous deaths of partners, friends and family. Such beliefs and experiences were not associable with any particular group of respondents, and the literature on death would suggest that some turn to the spiritual is quite common for the terminally ill, even when they have been agnostic, or at least hostile to organized religion, previously (e.g. Kubler-Ross, 1970). Some of the gay men did, however, describe some tensions between their religious beliefs and the predominating values in their gay social circles. The latter were often hostile to organized religion on the grounds that Christian denominations at the least are hypocritical on the issue of homosexuality (Anglicanism is the exemplar), if not openly homophobic (evangelical fundamentalists and puritanical Protestants). The same arguments would apply to militant forms of Islam.

The subjects who reported these tensions said that they saw their spiritual beliefs as a matter of individual conscience, and one man even perceived his church community as being more supportive to him as a gay man and PWA than his circle of gay friends and acquaintances. He had faced down criticisms of his religious beliefs:

Something was said and G turned round [another gay man in the drop-in at the Centre] and said, 'Oh, you're not going to turn religious on me, are you?' I said, 'No, I'm not going to turn religious, I have had my faith since I was four.'

New social worlds

Much of this individual refiguring of personal projects did not happen in a vacuum, through introspection and reading (though these may have played a part). The seeds were often sown through discussion with other HIV-positive people, and the most likely environment for this to occur in was a voluntary organization involved in social care: organizations such as Positively Women, Body Positive, the Centre, The Ace Project and Blackliners. All of these provided some form of drop-in facility, maybe as an adjunct to appointments for other services, where HIV-positive service users could meet and socialize with each other.

Beginning to use such an organization was described to me as itself problematic:

I'd come to the Centre twice before I built up the courage to go through the door. I knew once I entered this was who I'd be: someone with HIV, with other people with HIV. I couldn't face up to it. But now I'm really glad to have the Centre. It's made all the difference. (Gay man in his twenties)

And someone who had chosen not to use the Centre:

It's good they have places like that. But I wouldn't go. I just feel that if you see other people that it starts bringing it back you know, you end up with it probably getting worse.

Retrospectively, overcoming this inhibition was described as a very positive move, since organizations like the Centre subsequently played a major role in regenerating self-esteem and providing a new social world where some prior social withdrawal had been a common feature.

In one distinct group this generation of a social world was of supreme significance, since they were displaced in more than one sense. African women, especially those from Uganda, were often political refugees as well as HIV-positive. They may have had to flee their home country independently of partners and other family members; some had lost partners to AIDS before or after coming to Britain. They experienced cultural and economic isolation here, and tended to distance themselves from compatriots, and particularly members of their own ethnic groups, because of a strong stigma attaching to being HIV-positive. After their own diagnoses, referral to Positively Women and its support group at the Centre provided perhaps their only social network in Britain. The sense of support and belonging thus gained was repeatedly commented on.

> Yes, Positively Women have helped me a lot. They explain what all the leaflets mean. When we meet at the Centre I speak with people, including other Africans. I don't know other people in this country. I can get all the things I need at the Centre. (East African woman in her thirties)

The Centre provided a safe haven for such women, and often an opportunity to meet others from their own community who were similarly isolated, and whom they could trust to maintain confidentiality. The experience was not, however, without its problems. Most of these women were mothers with young children from whom the purpose of the Centre and the reasons their mothers were attending needed to be kept secret. With children of school age, various subterfuges had to be developed to maintain confidentiality, and in some cases this made women unwilling to continue coming to the Centre, even though it represented such an important social outlet.

Regaining a sense of social identity through an HIV/AIDS organization was not the prerogative of any particular group, though the form of the experience varied. Among the gay men was a core group (though with shifting membership) who lived and socialized locally, and for whom the Centre formed an adjunct to local gay social venues. They came to use the drop-in in a particular, familiar way, which did produce some tension with other user groups. I expand discussion of this theme in Chapter 4, arguing that identity and identity politics become a social, as well as individual tool, in the experience of negotiating shared use of HIV services. On an individual basis, though, organizations like the Centre broadly provided an environment for social reintegration. The sense of safety and confidentiality was crucial to this, of being amongst their own and the wise (cf. Goffman, 1963).

For the first six to seven months after diagnosis I was a recluse. I sat and drank in my room. I was rejected by my gay friends. I was very disappointed by their response to my diagnosis and I became bitter. They were the only people I really mixed with. I wished I'd gone to the Centre earlier and met others like me. I immediately felt less isolated when I did. I took solace from not being alone.

I would put on record that the Centre has been responsible for my new circle of friends, my flat and my belongings. Everything has come from the Centre and I'm grateful for this. (Gay man in his forties)

At the same time, relationships with organizations developed their own narratives, which were painful as well as productive. Participation could be a spur to more political involvement around HIV, or volunteering or seeking employment within the HIV sphere. Yet it could also mean seeing new friends become ill or die. With time, some respondents had begun to withdraw again, precisely because of the new losses they were experiencing. The ways that individual narratives develop therefore need understanding partially as a response to the contingencies of HIV, both in its effects on individual health and on the 'health' of someone's social network.

Summary

Cindy Patton has posed the question of whether PWA is more a policy device than an authentic self-identity (Patton, 1990, p. 8). This chapter has been an attempt to trace the range of ways in which HIV and AIDS influence aspects of self-identity. I have suggested that there are significant ways in which HIV and AIDS become identity markers, particularly where individuals become involved with HIV-related organizations and come to identify with others who are HIV-positive. Identification with HIV, and an assertion that being HIV-positive transcends other sources of difference, was a notable emergent theme in the study of the Centre, and this communal assertion of identity is discussed in the next chapter.

Processes of identity change for the individual can be usefully characterized in terms of Goffman's theories of stigmatization and the notion of biographical disruption in chronic illness. Some form of disruption of life script followed by a rewriting was common for my respondents, and similar to experiences with other forms of chronic illness (Bury, 1982; Robinson, 1988; Scambler, 1989). The content of this disruption varied considerably for individuals, and some of this variation can be identified with membership of particular groups. A positive HIV diagnosis had a significant impact on the sexual lives of many interviewees, and was described as a marker of difference. This sense of difference was linked with a concern over not infecting others: a study of the sexual health needs of HIV-positive gay and bisexual men similarly finds this sense of difference at the heart of many problems in relationships between sero-discordant male partners (Keogh *et al.*, 1995, pp. 37–8). And Elisa Sobo's study of disclosure of HIV-positive serostatus in New Mexico found similar concerns, regardless of the sexuality of focus group members (Sobo, 1995; Sobo *et al.*, 1995). However, the impact on self-identity of a positive diagnosis tended to have a particular significance for many of the gay men in our study, whose identities were built on membership of a sexualized culture in which sex talk was a significant part of everyday life. Ex-IDUs who were interviewed focused on the sense of separation connected with building a new life away from current drugs users. We had been unable to interview current users since there had been antagonism at the Centre between drugs users and other user groups. Again, the interplay of social and individual factors seems crucial to understanding how HIV affects identity.

Factors in the rebuilding of identity seem less linked with previous self-identity than the process of identity disruption, perhaps because the disruptive factor is held in common. So, the adoption of complementary therapies, volunteering for an HIV organization, or the exploration of spiritual ideas, were not correlated with any obvious group. This is interesting in that volunteering for HIV organizations among the general population *is* linked to identity factors: many of the volunteers are lesbians and gay men (Bebbington and Gatter, 1994; Kobasa, 1991; Lynn and Davis Smith, 1992). Again, this suggests that conceptualizing the personal experience of stigmatizing illness in terms of life scripts and biographical disruption is quite powerful. Our study does, however, indicate an area in which this approach is relatively weak. In discussing diagnosis and work, we saw how the experience of a middle-class professional in a public sector care organization could be quite different from that of someone unskilled or unemployed. These differences were manifold: illness could mean a bigger change of lifestyle for the former; yet provisions in relation to HIV in the workplace could also mean less disruption for the professional, even in the event of illness, depending on the ethos of the organization for which he or she worked. Thus the disruption and rewriting of the lifescript is to some extent materially determined, and is linked with social class and status as well as money. Access to services such as complementary therapies, except through some voluntary sector organizations such as the Centre and Immune Development Trust (IDT), depends on the ability to pay. Social class is rather a different identity factor to sexuality or gender, and is now unfashionable as an analytic concept. But it would seem that some account of the material constraints on identity, and attitudes and interests informed by social class, must form a complement to the postmodern or at least late modern account of identity, which tends to see it as a relatively unbounded project of the self in a pluralistic society. In this I agree with Steven Epstein: the development of identities is materially constrained (Epstein, 1987). Ways of responding to illness are similarly bounded.

Notes

1. The Helms amendment of 1987 effectively prevented the funding of gay education projects.
2. Further characteristics of this sample are detailed in Table 2.1 in Chapter 2.
3. Current medical research indicates that HIV begins multiplying in the body shortly after seroconversion, and that the immune system may be considerably damaged before the emergence of any clearly HIV-related illness. This might still be regarded as a latent period in that the subsequently diagnosed person may not have been aware of any problem at the time.
4. The active role of HIV-positive people in determining their treatment and care, and in promoting prevention and treatment activism, is discussed at length, in the American context, by Steven Epstein (1996).
5. *Continuum* persists as a journal which supports alternative understandings of AIDS.

4

Identity and Community: Social Practices and AIDS

The transformative power of HIV/AIDS for the gay community has been written about by many other writers. Activism on behalf of community has engendered a culture of caring not previously marked among gay men, at least not beyond their partners and closest friends (Kayal, 1993; Adam, 1992). In adopting such caring roles gay men have embraced hard, sometimes unpleasant work, seen as unmanly and traditionally associated with women (Wrubel and Folkman, 1997). At the same time an 'ownership' of HIV by gay men, a kind of double identity, has led to claims to authority to speak about HIV/AIDS on behalf of other gay men, and to the assumption of a self-evident community of need in relation to HIV/AIDS.

In a different direction, Dennis Altman argues that models for gay community AIDS activism developed in the West are being adopted by gay groups in South East Asia, particularly Malaysia, Thailand and Indonesia (Altman, 1994, p. 100). In the Philippines, a group of self-identified gay men (using the Western term 'gay') now sponsor work on HIV prevention as part of what they see as an emerging gay community (Tan, 1995, p. 86). Other culturally specific analyses have begun to consider how research on gay community may be incorporated into HIV prevention strategies. In Australia, Susan Kippax and colleagues have studied sexual behaviour and its connection with degrees of identification with gay community. Since community implies information networks, it is sensible to examine how these might be tapped into for distributing safer-sex messages, and drawing on research knowledge of how differ-ently situated gay men and other men who have sexual contact with men but don't identify as gay relate to their sexuality, in order to refine the notion of community (Kippax *et al.*, 1993).

The research instrument used in the Australian research was a closed-ended questionnaire. The picture of gay community identification and participation was built through developing rating scales of various respondent characteristics. For example, the level of attachment to gay community was judged in relation to answers to questions of the sort 'to whom have you revealed your gay identity?' and 'where do you spend your social life?' Although this project has clearly provided much infor-mation about gay community, I would argue that its findings are limited because community is not something that can be adequately understood through abstraction: it needs to be seen in operation. In this chapter I will demonstrate the use of an ethnographic approach to community, groun-ded in a perspective on what community is. To do this I need first to introduce the history of ways in which community has been conceptu-alized in the social sciences.

Conceptualizing community

Community is a key term in the lexicon of 1990s Britain. After the manifest individualism of 1980s Thatcherism, politicians claim they are trying to build community; that their opponents are set on tearing it apart. For Conservatism, community now replaces the state as the ideological site for support of the disadvantaged. Most obviously, this perspective lies behind the legislation for Care in the Community. This also is a site of ideological contest: several tragic incidents have been the focus for calling into question the wisdom of dealing with mental health problems in the 'community' rather than institutions.

The Conservative construction of community, like the family, is attacked from the political left as being unrealistic, and a cynical excuse for cutting public spending: both are fairytale phenomena premised on a bourgeois suburban fantasy of what life in Britain is really like. Yet community is very much part of the vocabulary of the political left, albeit in a progressively modified form. In New Labour's New Britain every-thing is of the people: the government, the party, the (late) Princess. Curiously, thinking of the Labour Party's history, this term now means 'all persons in Britain', a 'classless community', rather than the working class.

Community is not just a public, political term. Most of us speak at some point of belonging to various communities, both given and elective: black and Asian communities, the gay community, community associations, the professional community, the European community. Community thus means very different things, depending on context. To consider the significance of community for AIDS, we must start from a systematic exploration of its meanings in concrete social contexts. We must also analyse the relationship between community and identity, since they are overlapping concepts, and cannot be segregated where groups in late modernity (such as gay men) think of community in terms of lifestyle and identity.

Social science perspectives

There is an intractable problem with community, as stated in Peter Hamilton's foreword to Anthony Cohen's *The Symbolic Construction of Community* (1985). Social scientists have never been able to agree a definition of community. Reviewing usage, Sutton and Munson found 125 distinct definitions in 395 sociological publications between 1959 and 1976 (Sutton and Munson, 1976); Hamilton reports over 90 definitions by the 1950s (Hamilton, in Cohen 1985, p. 7). But this definitional confusion has to be weighed against the fact that people have a strong sense of belonging to communities and, if they feel this membership, it is real in its consequences.

Marx, reflecting ideas on the evolution of human society, saw community as a distraction from the *real* problem of class relations. It may once have existed, in the form of the primal horde, but it had become an irrelevance in bourgeois capitalist society; indeed it obscured economically exploitative relationships, was a form of ideology, and therefore of false consciousness. Furthermore, it is one of the few lay social terms that has exclusively positive connotations (Weeks, 1996, p. 71).

Such implicit evolutionism also informed much of the classic anthropology and sociology beginning in the mid-nineteenth century. Following Darwin (1859), the idea emerged that societies could be likened, metaphorically (though the metaphorical nature of the link was never properly acknowledged), to individual organisms. At any one time, the different parts of the organism were mutually interdependent: over time, the social organism evolved ever more complex institutions and processes. For example, Maine drew a distinction between societies in which relationships are conceived in terms of kin-based, ascribed hierarchies, as opposed to those (more advanced forms) in which relationships and interactions are negotiable on the basis of legal agreement: his classic distinction between 'status' and 'contract'. Tonnies proposed a slightly different distinction, between *Gemeinschaft* and *Gesellschaft*, the former being a society of intimacy and stability, the latter one where the individual is more atomized and interacts in discrete social contexts for different ends. Durkheim's parallel distinction was between mechanical and organic solidarity. All these approaches contained some attempt to account for the apparent differences between so-called small-scale traditional societies (past and present) and modern urban industrial nation states. They also implicitly carried a sentimentalized notion of community, a sense of human connectedness now lost in the anonymity of modernity.

It is important not to caricature these thinkers. Cohen is careful to emphasize that Durkheim, in particular, was not arguing a monolithic social evolutionism. Instead, he sought to illustrate the complexity of modern society by showing that mechanical and organic solidarity could exist side by side, even within the individual person, albeit perhaps in tension. He was arguing against a structural determinism that characterized vulgar Marxist analyses. Unfortunately, the mechanical/organic distinction became misread and overstated in the work of the highly influential Chicago School of anthropologists and sociologists in the mid-twentieth century. They projected Durkheim's distinctions onto the differences found between contemporary urban and rural North America. Thus rural life was communitarian, based on sustained face-to-face interaction, and involved an intimacy where people confronted one another as 'whole persons'. In contrast, the city demanded a fragmentation of social life where individuals interacted through 'roles' played out in diverse contexts. What was new was the value placed on this difference by the Chicago School. It was now the city that was the more desirable state of being. Urbanity was a more advanced form of human existence than custom and tradition-bound conservative rusticity.

For contemporary anthropologists, one of the most peculiar effects of this sociological tradition is the pre-eminence given to the idea of 'role'.

There appears to be a confusion between role as a sociological abstraction, and as a determining, empirical feature of real people in the modern world. As Cohen points out in *Self Consciousness*, we do not encounter one another as 'roles', as abstractions, but rather as complete selves and persons (Cohen, 1994, p. 7). This is obvious to common sense, but is also theoretically important in anthropology, which deals with the subject in culture, and is therefore averse to abstracting the person from the total social context in which he or she operates, or to dividing the person in a pseudopsychological fashion into a number of sub-personalities. This is important to the approach I will be taking here.

The main problems with the Chicago School way of thinking about community are twofold. First, it treats the nature of human association as being directly due to structural features of the size and scale of society, and asserts that fragmentation of the individual into progressively more specialized roles is necessitated by increasing size and complexity. It is, then, structurally deterministic, and, as Cohen says, possibly psychologically naive as it confuses the appearance of role-based social behaviour with what is actually occurring: the creative integration of these roles within the still intact human personality (Cohen, 1985, pp. 21–8). This confusion is evident again in the second problem: urbanization, according to the logic of the Chicago school, should spell the death of community. Empirically, this is clearly nonsense, since it is precisely in urban contexts that community has recently become a focus for social and cultural action. This is true for the gay community and AIDS in Britain, most obviously in London, but also in other urban centres such as Manchester and Brighton.

Both sociology and anthropology are increasingly using symbolic interactionist perspectives to explore the meanings of community. This is one way out of the impasse created by the Chicago School approach, since it allows community to be investigated inductively from the viewpoints of those who claim community membership, and makes no assumptions about communities being spatially bounded enumerable entities that embody, in Durkheim's term, some kind of mechanical solidarity (social linkage premised on interdependence and a high degree of face-to-face interaction, associated in Durkheim's original formulation with relatively undifferentiated pre-industrial societies). Secondly, a symbolic interactionist approach should avoid the idealization of community implicit in the assumption that community must be denied by urbanization. It is within a broadly symbolic interactionist approach that I situate the ethnographic methodology to be developed here.

Studying sexual communities

In the context of theorizing late modernity and the nature of urban life, a considerable body of work has appeared recently on communities premised on sexuality, particularly within lesbian and gay studies and interlocking areas of sociology and human geography (in practice the latter tends to mean work by sociologists and geographers who themselves are gay men or lesbians). Notably, the collection *Mapping Desire*, edited by David Bell and Gill Valentine (1995), takes forward our understanding of the geography of sexual community, while Jeffrey Weeks (1995, 1996), Mark Blasius (1994), Steven Epstein (1987) and others relate sexual community to identity politics and values.

The modern city provides a space in which subcultures can thrive. Sexual minorities colonize certain areas, socially and residentially (sometimes one without the other), typically in the inner city. Thus we have the idea of the 'gay ghetto', the Castro in San Francisco being the best-known example. Most of the literature on gay areas of cities has reflected this idea of ghettoization, along with gay gentrification, and has emanated from the United States (Herdt, 1992; Levine, 1979). *Mapping Desire* aimed to go beyond this position and, drawing on feminist thought and Queer theory, theorize precisely the ways in which spaces become sexualized (and vice versa). In this volume Larry Knopp proposed a framework for analysing sexuality and urban space that united subjectivity and lifestyle with an appreciation of the spatial divisions of activity in the city and the wider material forces that shape city life. He asked for an approach that takes into account the conflicting forces of class, gender, ethnicity and sexuality; his view of identity was a pluralist one, but, as a geographer, taking the city as the unit for conceptualization and analysis (Knopp, 1995).

The problem of spatial conflict in relation to identities is explored further by Myslik (1996) through the concept of territory. The term implies a sense of ownership, and is used to describe the relationship of place and social groups through relations of power. Significantly, for any analysis that attempts to include power as a dimension, Myslik intends 'territory' to refer to imagined as well as actual space, in other words to symbolic locations of community. Thus the relations between individuals, communities and spaces exist through social meanings as well as physical residence; they are socially constructed. In the context of sexual communities, spaces within cities may have a symbolic significance as 'gay' whether or not they can empirically be described as gay 'on the ground'. Following this analysis, gay communities are, at least in one sense, 'imagined communities' (Anderson [1983], cited in Mercer, 1995). Myslik goes on to suggest an interesting consequence of the symbolic dimension of sexual community. If an area is 'coded' as gay, this gives a sense of control and ownership to gay men. This may lead to a sense of safety in gay areas (Dupont Circle in Washington, DC, is cited as an example) when empirically such areas may be *relatively* dangerous because high concentrations of gay men in the inner city attract homophobic attentions. This is a good example of the reality and possible consequences of the imaginary.

Myslik's perspective embraces symbolic interactionism and social constructionism and, while focusing on urban space, complements my own perspective and related ones in sociology. The symbolic dimensions of community, in the sense of 'imagined' spaces or 'fictions' (see below) have become prominent in social constructionist analyses.

From a sociological rather than geographical perspective, Jeffrey Weeks summarizes contemporary thought on the idea of a sexual community in an article for *Soundings* (1996). He finds four key elements in sexual community, having first stated the case for seeing lesbian and gay communities as a critical case of late modern politicized identities:

- community as a focus of identity
- community as ethos or repository of values
- community as social capital[1]
- community as politics

Sexual communities for lesbians and gay men are first the relational outcome of a stigmatized minority identity, a search for their own and the wise (following Goffman). Historically, the possibility for such communities is only quite recent, the seeds sown by the scientific 'discovery' of the homosexual as a distinct kind of person in the second half of the nineteenth century (Foucault, 1978). Only since the late 1960s has sexual identity related to politics and community been a dominant motif

(Weeks, 1996, p. 75). This is a process of social construction in which the discredited assert their identity as a positive rather than a negative quality:

> Movements such as these are not simply expressing a pre-existing essence of social being. Identities and belongings are being constructed in the very process of organisation itself. (*ibid.*, pp. 75–6)

The idea of lesbian and gay community as ethos has been propounded by Mark Blasius. What he means by this is that communities premised on sexual identity can become the context for moral agency. Blasius sees coming out as a collective problematization of the self, a process of 'becoming' a political identity (Blasius, 1994, p. 180). This process is a search for 'communitas' through which actual communities may be built (see the discussion in Chapter 2).

Taking the example of gay community activism in response to AIDS, Weeks illustrates how community participation leads to an increase in social capital for the individual. By this he means that a variety of social skills can be drawn on in a collective endeavour that might otherwise not be available to the individual:

> Community based activities represent an attempt to gain control of the conditions of one's life, as again can be seen in the activities of the HIV/AIDS organisations. (Weeks, 1996, p. 80)

Sexual communities are often political in the way they subvert conventional politics, draw attention to themselves and lead to change. Groupings such as OutRage! obviously do this. Weeks defines contemporary lesbian and gay politics as moving from a moment of transgression to a moment of citizenship (*ibid.*, p. 82). The current emphasis is on campaigning for equal civil rights (e.g. Stonewall) rather than militant assertion of difference (on the whole, that is: OutRage! is an obvious exception).

These different senses of community overlap. Further, Weeks defines sexual communities as necessary fictions. Sexual communities do not necessarily exist in the strict sense of geographically bounded entities, or of empirically demonstrable social networks. Nonetheless, they are necessary fictions because, although imagined and invented, they enable and empower people through allowing the articulation of identity and can provide the substrate for actual political association and activity. I will return to this notion of community as necessary fiction in concluding this chapter, as it is useful in making sense of my ethnographic observations.

A methodological perspective

Community, as we have seen, is difficult to define lexically or as an analytical concept. Cohen suggests, instead, that we follow Wittgenstein in arriving at an understanding of community through its *use* rather than its lexical meaning. On this basis we might argue that, minimally, community implies that

> the members of a group of people (a) have something in common with each other, which (b) distinguishes them in a significant way from the members of other putative groups. 'Community' thus seems to imply simultaneously both similarity and difference. (Cohen, 1985, p. 12)

Community is thus a relational concept, and carries with it the implication of a boundary: that which separates one community from another and encapsulates its identity. Boundaries might be legal or geographical, but may equally be much less tangible, such as a sense of shared religious or sexual identity. Moreover, any one community may possess a number of bounding features; these features may be perceived differently by different individuals (on both sides of the boundary); and any individual may have a sense of belonging to several communities simultaneously. These commonsense observations lead Cohen to propose that we need to look at community primarily in terms of what it *means* to people. To do so gets away from the methodological limitation of structural determinism, and situates his approach within the paradigm shift since 1970 in anthropology (and some sociology) away from analysing culture and society in terms of form and function (adopted from the natural sciences) and towards thinking of them interpretatively (influenced by literary criticism, linguistics, semiotics and postmodernism more generally).

To look at meaning implies focusing on the symbolic dimension of community. What Cohen means by symbols is a set of ideas and principles that do not determine the thoughts of an individual, that is they are not rules, but nevertheless provide the framework within which cultural and social phenomena can be interpretable by individuals, so 'when we speak of people acquiring culture, or learning to be social, we mean that they acquire the symbols which equip them to be social' (*ibid.*, p. 16). The symbols of a community are most obvious in the way its boundaries are defined, both internally and in opposition to other perceived communities. These might be quite concrete, as in the rituals described extensively in the ethnographic literature: rites of passage, rituals demarcating the living from the dead, of gender segregation, and of life cycle stages, to name a few. Other symbolism, perhaps the majority, is far less marked and more intuitive. So words used by a community of itself, such as 'freedom', or of another community, such as 'fundamentalist', convey a greater abundance of meaning, and values, than their dictionary definitions would suggest.

The other important facet of symbols highlighted by Cohen is that they underspecify their meanings to individuals: individuals always supply part of their meanings. Thus gender, age, death and so on are all symbols of a group of people who share the same language and participate in the same symbolic behaviours surrounding them, but the exhaustive meaning of each symbol is mediated by the 'idiosyncratic experience of the individual' (*ibid.*, p. 14). Some social categories are more fixed in their meanings than others, but those that are most open to interpretation are also those that are most beset with ambiguous symbolism: this is true of community itself.

> As a symbol, it is held in common by its members; but its meaning varies with its members' unique orientations to it. In the face of this variability of meaning, the consciousness of community has to be kept alive through the manipulation of its symbols. (*ibid.*, p. 15)

This approach allows us to account for quite discrepant ideas within community by persons who would nevertheless agree they all belong to the same community. What the approach is much weaker at is specifying and analysing the processes of contestation of meaning within community: whose definitions become accepted, how, and why? There is a tendency in much current identity politics literature to celebrate difference without problematizing it, to resort to a kind of flaccid pluralism (discussed in Seidman, 1996; see especially Gamson, 1996). The rejection of class-based and other materialist analyses seems to have been accompanied by an abandoning of any attempt to take power seriously as a relevant analytic concept.

If the spatial metaphor of boundary is accepted, it might also be appropriate to think in terms of landscapes within boundaries. A community will contain hills and valleys, rivers and plains. How these appear will depend on the perspective of an individual situated in time and space within the landscape. However, to continue the metaphor, this landscape is not immutable. There will be earthquakes and flash floods as well as tranquil days. The landscape will erode; rivers will change their courses over time, yet the boundary may remain intact.

We can begin then to look at the nature of gay community in relation to AIDS by applying Cohen's symbolic analysis while also needing an adequate account of the power dimension of community. In developing such an analysis I will make use of the activities and proclamations of gay activists working in the HIV/AIDS field, and data from individual interviews and group meetings in the HIV/AIDS organization I was involved in evaluating. In relation to other perspectives on community and identity described in this chapter, it must be borne in mind that my focus is on the articulation of community as a symbol by people who claim community membership: it is not about spatial, residential communities, nor the sexual aspects of gay community (social or spatial).

The Oratory

In a deliberate polemic in the London listings magazine *Time Out* (Gay section, 8–15 February 1995), Mark Simpson wrote about what he called the 'AIDS Clergy' and their unholy trinity of 'one disease, one cause, one response'. This is an attack on what might be described as the orthodox position on AIDS among gay AIDS activists with the highest public profile in Britain. Chief target of Simpson's venom is Edward King, who has written extensively in the gay press on AIDS issues (most obviously as AIDS Editor for the *Pink Paper* in the mid-1990s) as well as working for the National AIDS Manual and being a director of Gay Men Fighting AIDS. The substance of Simpson's salvo appears to be an indictment of those who set themselves up as the arbiters of AIDS knowledge on behalf of the gay community, who support the hypothesis that HIV is the sole cause of AIDS and label those who demur from this view as heretics. Some personal, if peripheral, involvement in this circle suggests to me that an amount of personality clashing and character assassination is involved as well, albeit under the guise of fighting an important battle for the gay community.

The point in raising this example is to begin to suggest that the public debates about gay community and AIDS are always more than descriptive and practical. They are ideological also. They are about making claims, which may have consequences.

A relevant starting-point for examining gay perspectives on community and AIDS is Edward King's *Safety in Numbers* (1993). His text is aimed specifically at tracing the role of gay men in relation to the HIV epidemic in the West and to use this material to argue for greater resource dedication to gay men's sexual health. He recounts the empirical details of the epidemiology of HIV since 1981 and argues strongly that informal peer education in gay communities was a major influence for containing HIV in the mid to late 1980s, particularly in Britain (King, 1993, pp. 37–84). The argument continues that with the advent of government health education campaigns aimed at the general population (and specifically *not* at gay men) and a dulling of activism among gay men after the initial shock of AIDS, the incidence of HIV was able to increase again at the beginning of the 1990s (this position is supported by others, such as van den Hoek, van Griensven and Coutinho, 1990). King's argument tends to be selective in its use of empirical research findings, and it would, for example, be very difficult to prove the assertion that the British government's active inattention to gay men's health needs has 'had considerable harmful consequences for the sustenance of safer sex among gay men' (King, 1993, p. 188; no evidence is cited), especially when set against the claim that it was largely a sense of mutual responsibility among gay men that held the virus in check in the earlier years.

Whatever the merits or faults of King's argument, how can we see community as symbolically constructed in it? The idea of peer education implies a sense of connectedness and mutual responsibility, which reflects Cohen's minimal definition of community. It is not simply that the community's members are the same, but that this sameness evokes a sense of common cause where AIDS is concerned. And this common cause is delineated in and against a boundary separating gay men from all others. 'The government' and 'gay men' are clearly constructed as mutually exclusive categories.[2] Stigma, linked with the triad of AIDS, sexuality and death, is a dominant symbol around which gay community coheres.

This analysis is supported by Philip Kayal's portrayal of volunteerism in GMHC in New York. Kayal, writing from the explicit subject positions of a gay man and sociologist, argues that volunteerism among gay men in relation to AIDS can only be understood through the relation between subjectivity and community. Certain structural features of AIDS have forced gay men (and not others) to action. AIDS literally attacks the fabric of gay community because of how it is most often transmitted; this is not so for heterosexuals. Most strikingly, Kayal argues that AIDS has informed gay identities by demanding participation in, and transformation of, community. Gay men of often high social status have turned altruistically to support others with whom they are connected only by being gay, and to perform sometimes physically unpleasant caring tasks, culturally associated in the West with women (and thus not highly valued). Rooted in a history of gay activism, the gay response to AIDS, according to Kayal, can be seen as both a reaction to institutionalized homophobia (Kayal, 1993, p. 29) and a journey towards overcoming internalized homophobia (*ibid.*, p. 96). Gay men, whether HIV positive or not, volunteer for PWAs because they are all members of a 'community for rejected others seen as the extended self' (*ibid.*, p. 110).

Counterposing King and Kayal suggests two avenues for enquiry. A first-order analysis might consider how community is symbolically constructed in gay voices on AIDS. A secondary analysis would then move on to the historical effects of AIDS on the discourses of gay community – the transformative process highlighted by Kayal. Although both forms of analysis have not so far been combined in a single longitudinal research project, my aim here is to make a case for this approach through a mosaic of existing accounts. My sources are of two major kinds: statements and writings from those who claim to represent gay community (following King); and my own empirical research at the Centre, looking at the negotiation of community at a 'grass-roots' level.

Naming and claiming: who we are

In the mid-1980s, when the British government began to take notice of AIDS, many (self-identifying) gay men working in the field supported the notion of HIV prevention campaigns aimed at the general public. Their intention was to avoid the stigmatization of AIDS as a 'gay disease'. A corollary was the development of the neologism 'Men Who Have Sex With Men' (MWHSWM, MSM and other variants). It was widely accepted that a large but covert population of men had sex with other men but did not outwardly (or even inwardly, in some cases) identify as gay. They were at risk from HIV, but not likely to come into contact with the peer support already recognized within the 'out' gay community.

MSM is a problem term. It is an analytic description that has no real referents in terms of lived identities. Since the beginning of the 1990s this problem has been at the core of an ideological battle over community, identity and gay men's alignment with HIV and AIDS. As Simon Watney put it:

> This supposed group has special significance in academic research since it is thought of as the main route of possible HIV transmission from 'the gay community' to 'innocent' heterosexuals ... In other words, the category of MSMs is little more than a reconceptualization of the earlier concept of the 'bridging group', imagined as a Trojan horse full of 'AIDS carriers' inside the 'heterosexual community'. (Watney, 1993, p. 23)

MSM has come to be seen by gay activists as a distraction from the real problem that gay men are denied the HIV prevention and care resources that they deserve – a process termed the 'degaying' of AIDS (see King, 1993, for a fuller account). The reaction has been a call for the 'regaying' of AIDS, and it is this that has provoked a mushrooming of arguments about the nature of gay identity and its link with community. Thus, during the 1990s, shifts in government policy and their reception by gay activists can be seen as material causes for a changing emphasis on the nature and role of gay community for AIDS. This is the historical framework in which more detailed debates need to be inscribed.

Part of the argument for the regaying of AIDS is that it is out gay men, active on the gay scene, and who identify as members of the gay community, who are at highest risk of infection with HIV in Britain (King, 1993, p. 264). Discussions of this 'group' by gay activists give the impression that its membership is self-evident. No clear statements are made about who precisely counts as a member. Gay community is a social category variable in meaning, and, following Cohen, we might expect it to be hedged around by ambiguous symbolism.

Findings from empirical research on HIV prevention point up the partiality of some of the activist arguments. The MESMAC Project (Men Who Have Sex with Men – Action in the Community), funded by the Health Education Authority in the early 1990s, sought to establish a number of educational programmes around England which included outreach and agency work, and was guided by the philosophy of Community Development (Deverell, 1992; Prout and Deverell, 1995). The evaluation of MESMAC found a complex relationship between sexual identities, other identities, and sexual behaviours (as discussed in Chapter 2). Among the clients of the project, ethnic minority men often had no attachment to the identity 'gay', or even actively rejected it as Western, white, or middle-class. Race would loom larger than sexuality in their self-perceptions, and the meanings of and attachments to family were often qualitatively different from those of white gay men. Among the project workers, although it was commonly asserted that gay men were best placed to work with gay men, there was ambiguity about working with non-gay-identified men who were having sexual contact with other men. Someone bearing gay identity signifiers (dress, speech, mannerisms) might be avoided by MSMs who rejected sexuality labels. Furthermore, labels could be confusing: outreach workers made assumptions about the kinds of men they were approaching in public spaces which didn't always prove correct (Prout and Deverell, 1995, p. 73).

Similar findings have been reported in Australian research. A study of men using public sex environments ('beats') found that non-gay-identifying men often sought sexual partners in mainstream 'straight' nightclubs as well as the beats, and didn't see themselves as having any identity premised on sexuality (Davis, Klemmer and Dowsett, 1991). The authors concluded that what might be termed behavioural bisexuality needs to be seen as contingent on situations, settings and sexual possibilities, rather than the expression of a social and sexual identity (see also Sigma Research, 1996, for similar findings in Britain). In relation to this problem of identity, it is germane that some of the workers and clients of the MESMAC project actively embraced the MWHSWM terminology as descriptively accurate and not bearing the symbolic load of a rejected identity (Prout and Deverell, 1995, p. 215). This contradicts Simon Watney's argument, and also fits in with the general thesis of this book that identities have to be understood as constantly in process of development, and as strategic and contested entities.

Gay activists have recognized that gay community is a nebulous concept, in that its members are very diverse in respects other than their sexuality. But they wish to promote the clearly defensible argument that a sense of belonging to community may have positive results in limiting the spread of HIV: people within community are more likely to be part of informal HIV information networks, and to have reasonable self-esteem about their sexuality and sexual practices. Calling for more resources and targeted HIV prevention strategies implies, however, that gay community must be actively engaged by outside forces (such as the Department of Health), and energized from within. To this end, activists *are* trying to define the nature of gay community and how best it might be engaged by health promotion.

This defining process itself must be seen in historical context. In the 1970s gay activism in Britain was tied explicitly to the politics of the left. This heritage persists in diverse groups (Stonewall, CHE and others) which campaign for representation and civil rights of gay men and lesbians. More recent groups, such as OutRage! and ACT UP (AIDS Coalition to Unleash Power), have a different agenda. ACT UP originated in the United States, and OutRage! in Britain was founded on similar lines, which is significant. Though civil rights are a prominent issue in the United States, they are couched in terms of individual self-determination, identity, and lifestyle linked to identity (i.e. identity politics), rather than in relation to a materialist, class-based politics. With the current crisis in the left–right divide in Britain (perhaps most obvious in Blairism) and the fact that gay identity is not fully congruent with class politics (even if most out gay men and lesbians lean to the left), it is unsurprising that the focus of gay community activism is shifting towards the American model (a positioning explicit, for example, in the work of Simon Watney; see *Practices of Freedom*, 1994).

I saw, I conquered, I came

The framing by activists of gay identity and community has recently tended to be in terms of community of sexual interest:

> In reality the lesbian and gay community has always been a network of communities, primarily split between a political community which pursues an ideal of political power and

representation, and the communities of the night, which encompass the genuine diversity which political activists seek to represent. (Alcorn, 1992)

'Communities of the night' is a phrase potent in imagery of danger, desire and (perhaps) romance, reclaiming 'the twilight world of the homosexual' in positive terms. I would argue that it obscures as much as it reveals. Sexual object orientation is not in itself a sufficient condition for an identity, nor even practices related to that orientation. The question of interest is how the 'communities of the night' idea constructs sexualities and what effects this has.

Behaviour does not 'contain' meaning intrinsically; rather, it is found to be meaningful by an act of interpretation: we 'make sense' of what we observe. (Cohen, 1985, p. 17)

Community of sexual interest casts the defining feature of gay community as sexual contact: semen as social adhesive, if you like. In the context of HIV this is a useful symbol since it suggests a deliberately blurred boundary, including all out gay sexually active men, but also any man they have sex with who doesn't identify in this way.[3] Because HIV is mainly transmitted sexually between gay men, gay activists now see reaching the 'communities of the night' as a high priority; and since these communities are defined as being *about* sex, eroticizing safer sex is an appropriate mode of health promotion. Beyond this, their emphasis indicates a preoccupation with sexual freedom as an aim of gay identity politics. While writers such as Kayal have focused on the altruistic aspects of community enhanced by AIDS, and a growing attention to intimate relationships among gay men, activist positions tend towards an almost exclusive sex positivity. If anything, discussion of intimacy and caring has been derided on the grounds that HIV prevention is the overriding necessity, and ideas of intimacy and romance can lead to complacency about safer sex (Hardy, 1990), while also mimicking heterosexist moralities of sexuality. At least, this was the case at the time of our research. Only in the mid to late 1990s has there been a shift towards a focus on HIV within long-term monogamous and non-monogamous relationships, and to appreciating the significance of the meanings of different kinds of relationships to those involved in them, to the refining of HIV prevention. Such changes have accompanied political and medical developments over the past few years, which I discuss in greater detail in Chapter 6.

Attached to the activist concern with community of sexual interest is a set of arguments about the distribution of resources, and the appropriate role of out gay men in relation to other men having sex with men. Out gay men on the commercial scene are argued to be at highest risk of HIV because of the number of sexual partners they have and their likelihood of experiencing contexts in which unsafe sex is possible (King, 1993, p. 248). These men deserve health promotion resources from government, but these are most effectively delivered by gay men for gay men: the MSM strategy is alienating and seen as clinical and authoritarian by out gay men (*ibid.*, p. 204). The fluid boundary between these and other men does, however, provide a rationale for including non-gay-identifying men in health promotion. Hard-to-reach, sexually marginal men connect with out gay men sexually. Gay men are therefore the best placed people to convey safer sex information to them. A more radical version of this argument maintains that since a proud gay identity is most likely to sustain safer sex through high self-esteem, sexually marginal men are best served by bringing them into the gay community, by creating the conditions in which an out gay identity can be adopted. This is among the aims of the campaigning organization GMFA, and has also been argued for by Simon Watney (1993, pp. 24–6), among others.

Asserting community through difference

The London Gay Men's HIV Workers' Forum (an informal network of statutory and voluntary sector workers and activists) met in March 1995 to discuss 'Regaying Revisited',[4] a meeting which I attended as a participant. The group recognized that since the *National AIDS Manual* (*NAM*), GMFA, the THT and North West Thames Regional Health Authority HIV Project had drawn attention to the dearth of work targeted to gay men's needs in Britain in 1992 (King *et al.*, 1992) the situation had considerably improved. In two studies commissioned by the *National AIDS Manual*, 84 per cent of service-purchasing health authorities were found to identify gay, bisexual, and other MSM as a target group. The proportion was lower in local authorities, though this was due in part to a greater emphasis on generic (rather than HIV/AIDS specific) services and structurally different priorities for prevention and care when compared with the health service (*NAM*, 1994a, 1994b). The discussion following presentation of these reports focused on the need to avoid complacency. Respondents had identified targeting of gay men for services but did not describe, either qualitatively or quantitatively, what this commitment meant operationally.

Perhaps, one health promotion worker suggested, we had presented a simplistic picture of gay community to expedite the targeting of gay men. Perhaps now it was appropriate that core gay identified men, both as workers in the HIV/AIDS field and targets of this work, should act as the conduits to others whose identity and participation in a community of sexual interest were more problematic. This is a diluted version of the GMFA argument described above.

At this point in the debate a research worker involved in the evaluation of the health promotion initiatives of the previous speaker's organization challenged his interpretation. The evaluation research had shown that groups of men identifiable by different criteria (all of whom had sex with other men in some context) were often discrete populations having no contact, nor wish for contact, with each other.

This interchange encapsulates a key problem in looking at gay community and HIV/AIDS. The insights of a piece of social scientific research, aimed at helping improve health promotion, contest the suggestions of an activist/worker whose aims are the same. The activist has an agenda that may be classed as having political and ideological dimensions. But precisely because of these dimensions, he may at a later date prove the researcher wrong. The GMFA/Watney argument is, critically, one for social change, for enabling people to find their identities, identities that are unfairly stigmatized. Identities, and senses of belonging in community, can be transformed by cultural and political programmes. We are back with the point that identities are unstable and contestable in the late modern or postmodern world: they are not the innate and inalienable essence of a transcendent self.

Ethnography in an AIDS service organization

The various threads of this chapter can now be pulled together by exploring a case study. This will provide a concrete context for applying the methodological and theoretical perspective I have been developing.

The case concerns the social support facilities of the voluntary sector ASO, the Centre, discussed in terms of individual experience in Chapter 3. The Centre had been opened in an inner-city area of South London, in 1989, after a group of professionals working in the health service and local government, together with some HIV-affected local people, recognized a need for social care services in a non-clinical environment. This group were determined to endorse a non-discriminatory service provision environment for everyone affected by HIV, regardless of gender, race, ethnicity, sexual orientation, or probable route of HIV transmission. At that time they were seeking to counter widespread prejudice and misunderstanding of HIV and AIDS in British society.

This concern was made explicit in various ways when the Centre finally opened. Staff dedicated to working with ethnic minority groups and injecting drugs users were appointed early on in the Centre's history. Service information sheets for service users emphasized 'equal opportunities' for all in receiving services. All these expressions of non-discrimination were symbolized in the organization's letter heading, which depicted an open door admitting sunlight. The staff and directors (which the founding group had become) spoke frequently of the Centre's open-door ethos: all users of the organization (including staff and volunteers) were to be treated equally, the minimum of data were to be collected on service users (since monitoring was perceived as intrusive and likely to compromise trust), and all service users were to be regarded *as if* the only issue relevant to their presence at the Centre was HIV (that they were HIV-positive themselves or strongly affected by HIV as a partner or carer of someone else). The Centre shared an ethos and ideology with other voluntary sector HIV/AIDS organizations which had some of their roots in identity politics and social movements: a focus on user empowerment (with values of non-discrimination and non-stigmatization), a belief in the utility of alternative or complementary therapies, and a critical perception of the 'expert' status of the medical profession (Bennett and Ferlie, 1994, pp. 125–6).

Until a year or so after the Centre had opened, the open-door ethos seemed to be widely upheld by the service users themselves. They saw themselves as linked to each other through HIV status and, at least while in the building, not divided according to other criteria. There was an active ideology of harmony: the Centre was to be a haven.

During the course of our research fieldwork various changes occurred, which resulted in the 'community' of the Centre becoming much more divided, changes which can be seen in the context of the bureaucratization and routinization of voluntary associations more generally. Theorists of organizational behaviour and culture see bureaucratization as an inevitable feature of the incorporation of 'grassroots' organizations within larger state agencies such as the NHS, and suggest that such processes will occur even where voluntary agencies remain independent if they are in a dependent position (Bennett and Ferlie, 1994, Ch. 3). Such change has been described as occurring at the THT during its formative years (Schramm-Evans, 1990).

The first influence for change in the ethos of the Centre was a major shift in the funding environment for its services. Since opening in 1988 the bulk of service funding had come from the Department of Health, but with the NHS and Community Care Act (1990) came the requirement for services to be provided through potentially competitive contractual arrangements, replacing the earlier system of block grants from the Department of Health to voluntary sector organizations. This was the key feature of the introduction of a quasi-market system within the health service, which split the purchasing of services from their provision. A National Audit report at this time had found that existing financial data and monitoring systems within the NHS were inadequate, and would need considerable improvement if contracting was to work efficiently (National Audit Office, 1991). The pressures for accountability were particularly acute in the case of HIV/AIDS services since AIDS, uniquely at this time, attracted ring-fenced funding, i.e. funding guaranteed to be used for a stated purpose, which cannot be redirected to other ends at a later date.

A related pressure for change towards looking like a conventional service provision organization was the need to appear respectable, efficient and professional in order to be credible with funders. In common with other ASOs, the Centre had a very strong gay presence among its staff, directors, volunteers and service users. In the context of the early 1990s this was played down in concert with the general trend to 'degaying', but also to avoid the stigma that might attach to a gay community organization, or the suspicion that professional roles might become subordinate to sexual interests and community identification (see Cain, 1994, for a similar analysis of a Canadian ASO).

One effect of these changes was that organizations such as the Centre ended up monitoring much more closely the volumes of services provided to identified categories of client: this was both to make accurate estimates of demand, required for making funding bids, and to show *ex post facto* that money received had indeed been used to meet the needs of the local HIV-affected population. Ironically, the equal opportunities requirements of different funders, and of the Centre internally, meant that much more information had to be collected that distinguished one HIV-positive person from another.

The other major and material influence for change in the service provision ethos of the Centre was that as the Centre gained a reputation for the quality of its services and, sadly, the number of local HIV-positive cases increased, the numbers of people wishing to use its facilities were rapidly increasing, so both time and space soon became limiting factors in service provision.

On the introduction of these structural changes we began to notice changes in the way that service users articulated their interests: specifically, that interests began to be expressed in identity terms, particularly gay identity. According to the minimal statistics kept by the Centre from the outset, some 61 per cent of service users in September 1990 were gay men, 15 per cent women, and 9 per cent black or minority ethnic members (Centre cumulative service user statistics). These abstract proportions did not change significantly over the following year, but the real persons thus labelled entered an ideological arena where identity and community were concerned.

The social life of the Centre revolved around a drop-in area where visitors could socialize and have meals. It operated on an open-access basis to begin with, except for one evening per week for women only. This was uncontroversial, but the pressures for monitoring, together with time and space restrictions, led the Centre's management to decide that more services would need to be targeted in future, including the drop-in. A drop-in session for black people was planned, given that service uptake by this group was relatively low, and problems with staff coverage of drop-in led to an overall reduction of drop-in hours (there were no dedicated drop-in staff at this time).

A core, articulate group of gay men who had come to know each other through the drop-in began to see these service changes as an erosion of service access *for gay men as a group*. They felt subjected to some of the discrimination against gay men experienced in the world outside the

Centre, and indeed were heard to relate their experience at the Centre to the wider discourse in the gay press and AIDS activist organizations about the 'degaying of AIDS'. A combative atmosphere began to develop at the Centre, evidenced by a number of incidents, in which a clear, strong, self-promotional voice among gay men began to be heard.

At a volunteers' meeting at which service changes were discussed, the following views were expressed:

Gay male transport volunteer: 'I'm getting the impression that drivers are being hived off to provide lifts only for the women on women's night. I know the women need resources as well, but it's really beginning to feel as if things are being taken away from gay men, when we're the group who's been most affected by HIV over the past ten years.'

Female transport volunteer: 'I disagree with that. Women have always had poorer access to services, so there's a need to balance things out a bit.'

Female volunteer manager: 'I think there's been a misunderstanding. Lifts are given on the basis of driver availability, and the building is a women-only space on Wednesday nights anyway.'

At other times, gay men argued with each other over lines of identity divisions, simultaneously acknowledging and denying difference. For example, in the drop-in:

Black gay man: 'I've just been to a meeting for people of colour. They just didn't want to discuss HIV. I think we need a centre for black people who are HIV-positive now.'

White gay man no. 1: 'We shouldn't do that, it would be a kind of apartheid.'

White gay man no. 2: 'It's not being grown up about the issue to do that. Everyone with HIV is in the same position. It doesn't matter about race.'

White gay man no. 1: 'It would be stupid to do that anyway as there are not enough resources to go round as it is.'

Note that there was no perception among the white men here that their statements might be racist: in this context they saw being HIV-positive and gay as the relevant issues. In HIV prevention research there have been similar reports of the invisibility of race, of it being subsumed within HIV. Thus, one of the black workers interviewed for the MESMAC evaluation stated:

> My own experience of talking to white gay men is that black feelings are marginalised and dismissed. [It's either] 'We're all gay, we all feel the same', or they've never thought about it. (in Prout and Deverell, 1995, p. 115)

A key incident occurred at the consultative committee, which had been set up to allow dialogue between staff, volunteers and service users about how the Centre was being run and the direction of service development.

> *Women's evening service user representative:* 'Several of the women feel awkward bringing their children in here because of the safer sex posters on the walls.'

> *Gay male service user no. 1:* 'Are they complaining about the fact the posters are explicit, or that they show gay couples?'

> *Female volunteer:* 'Only some of the posters show gay couples. I think the mothers are more concerned about sexual material generally.'

> *Gay male service user no. 2:* 'I don't believe that. It's not as if it's pornographic. I think these people are just being homophobic.'

> *Female volunteer no. 2:* 'If they are being homophobic that's not acceptable. It's their own problem if they feel awkward coming in the building.'

> *Gay male service user no. 3:* 'Look, if it matters that much, why not take the posters down just for the women's evening? But I still feel offended because it sounds like homophobia.'

Female volunteer no. 3: 'I think the most important thing is that people need educating about HIV, and that includes children. Trying to protect children from safer sex images is misplaced morality.'

Women's evening representative: 'But the women still won't want to come here during the day if the posters are up.'

The outcome of this debate was an uneasy compromise that the posters be removed on women's evening. The management of the Centre felt they had to respond to accusations of homophobia, even in the absence of any concrete evidence. Similar tensions between differing identities and organizational priorities are reported for a community-based ASO in Canada (Cain, 1994). In this case the argument again revolved around openness. The workers in the organization felt that open discussion of sexuality was a public duty, but dispute arose over sexually explicit HIV prevention materials:

> these posters concerned some members of the board, who had received a complaint about their gay content. The board eventually decided to display in public view only those AIDS education posters which are unlikely to offend people; sexually explicit posters would only be hung in a back office, away from general view. The board decided, in effect, to conceal the stigma symbols. (Cain, 1994, p. 55)

In the wake of all these events many gay men using services at the Centre came to identify as a community with common needs under threat. Reactively, other groups began to 'commune' around identities. Women who were mothers, and others who supported them, campaigned for a more child-friendly and child-safe environment. A sizeable group of refugees from Eastern Africa (particularly Uganda) were recognized as having particular cultural needs quite different from gay men.

The appearance of a strong gay identity within the Centre was not born of nothing: the individuals who constituted the group brought their own histories of marginalization and oppression. Notably, unlike Kayal's GMHC volunteers, a high proportion of them were working-class and experiencing other forms of stress, such as unemployment. They were more likely to express their demands in confrontational ways than their more bourgeois counterparts. Nevertheless, what might previously have been a partly dormant sense of self and community was enabled to emerge in a historical process in which structural, institutional pressures can be identified as playing a role. The circumstances described may have had unique consequences at the Centre, but the ethnography indicates the kinds of factors that may be significant to the formation and transformation of identities more generally. At the same time, given that all ASOs were affected by the Community Care legislation, it is likely that some of what occurred at the Centre has been closely paralleled elsewhere.

Although I have focused on the strategic use of identity by service users and volunteers here, it is important to note that the phenomenon has been prevalent in the setting up and running of ASOs, and at all levels within such organizations. The general environment of the British response to AIDS (see Chapter 6) was one in which a culture of equal opportunities played an important role in the 1980s and early 1990s, when funding for AIDS services was relatively abundant. In particular, gay men in influential positions within health and social services were able to use their identities as levers for securing funding. In a different piece of research in which I was involved, one of the men responsible for setting up the HIV care services of an inner London borough stated quite candidly:

Yes, I used being an openly gay man to manipulate the situation. I knew they wouldn't have dared say no at the time. I was even able to bypass most of the bureaucratic obstacles by being 'in your face' with my colleagues.

Community in HIV prevention and care

The gay men I have described were gay men before they started using the Centre. It would be foolish to claim that sexual identity *in the sense of sexual orientation* was changed in any significant way by participation in the life of the Centre. Rather, I have attempted to illustrate the validity of seeing an identity strongly founded on sexuality as something larger than sexual orientation, something which may be transformed historically through specific sets of material and ideological pressures.

Following the discussion of nascent 'HIV-positive' and 'PWA' identities in Chapter 3, I have tried to show here how fragile such an identity is in relation to gay community and other situated senses of community. The analysis has been applied to gay men, but could be directed elsewhere. Nevertheless, these identity processes have a special character for gay men in relation to HIV/AIDS, a point to be developed further in the next chapter, which compares experiences of HIV/AIDS with other chronic illnesses.

The kinds of tensions I have illustrated between groups at the Centre have been analysed in a different sense by Joshua Gamson (1989, 1996). His interest is in new social movement theory (derived from Habermas) and its applicability to community responses to HIV/AIDS. Social movements of the 1960s were premised on social divisions such as class and gender. In the 1980s and 1990s the groups mobilizing around AIDS have done so predominantly in relation to lifestyle politics (he characterizes gay political identification in lifestyle terms), though some other groups are aligned in more 'traditional' groupings (thus, in Britain, we have had black HIV/AIDS organizations such as Blackliners and the Black HIV/AIDS Network). Gamson asserts that these different forms of group identification interact differently with the politics of AIDS activism, making it difficult for a 'rainbow coalition' to survive in HIV/AIDS organizations, in spite of protestations of 'needing to pull together to defeat the greater evil'. There are further contradictions to be found in the fact that gay men need to 'own' AIDS in order to secure resources, yet need to repudiate the stigma attaching to AIDS.

Gamson suggests that social movement theory is moving away from rational actor models towards seeing collective identity as itself a process or even an end in itself:

> Collective identity, in this model, is conceptualized as 'a continual process of recomposition rather than a given,' and 'as a dynamic, *emergent* aspect of collective action.' (Gamson, 1996, p. 398, citing Schlesinger, 1987, p. 237, original emphasis)

If we take Gamson's suggestion together with Cohen's theoretical perspective discussed at the beginning of this chapter, we see that both individual and group identities are historical products of interaction, literal and symbolic.

I offer a more detailed examination of Gamson's theoretical position in an article for *Social Science and Medicine* (Gatter, 1995). Here I suggest his work as a valuable complement to understanding the wider forces shaping particular instances of community conflict, and how and why these may remain unresolvable. His analysis, however, focuses on ACT UP, an in-your-face activist organization in the United States that has used public spaces and theatrics to make its points. The context, then, is quite different from a caregiving organization with formal divisions of rights and responsibilities.

Another useful theoretical formulation is Cain's analysis of the Canadian ASO. He frames his analysis of internal organizational tensions and change in terms of stigma: that the organization was set up to counter stigma, and that the stigmatized identities of those involved in the organization (gay men, injecting drugs users, black people) profoundly shaped how the organization responded to the external environment and negotiated internal differences. Drawing on Goffman, Cain sees the history of the ASO in terms of the management of stigma (Cain, 1994). Cain argues that stigma is the main culprit for a failure to build and sustain political alliances across identity divisions, whereas Gamson looks to the influence of discourses and fields of knowledge, to constellations of power/knowledge. In the end the two analyses are complementary, though framed in very different terms.

With less theoretical ambition, the ethnographic examples I have described in this chapter have helped illustrate how community and community membership are used strategically in achieving individual aims. Yet this is not to deny that community has some reality also at a group level. Community and identity within community involve a constant dialectic between the individual and the group, and I have shown how material imperatives (in this case HIV care resources) may constrain and direct relations between individuals, expressed identities, and communities.

On a practical level, claims made in group and communitarian terms within HIV/AIDS organizations need very careful scrutiny. Organizational decisions about service provision in Britain's current culture of citizenship and service user input requires organizations to listen to their users. Although I am not suggesting that a social constructionist analysis of the sort used here will answer immediate policy questions on how resources should be distributed (either generally or in particular organizations), I think it is clear that 'needs' are not things 'out there' waiting to be discovered. They are, in part at least, ideological productions. As productions of socially constructed communities they have a symbolic dimension related to the power to make claims. Needs are, therefore, both 'imagined' and 'fictional', though this does not mean they are not real. Their reality in any visceral, literal sense can only ever be incomplete.[5]

Notes

1. Social capital is an increasingly fashionable term, politically and academically. It derives metaphorically from the concept of economic capital. Unfortunately, it is often not rigorously defined, and is used very differently by different commentators. Its status as a rigorous analytical concept remains dubious.
2. This is not in any way to deny that gay sexuality has been highly stigmatized in Britain; nor to suggest that within politics it has always been the Conservative party that is most vexed by, and duplicitous about, homosexuality.
3. This position still excludes ways of describing the identities of two non-gay-identifying men having sex.
4. For a social science analysis of the events surrounding the 'degaying' and 'regaying' of AIDS see Weeks *et al.*, 1996.
5. These comments relate to HIV/AIDS voluntary organizations and social care. I would not make such a strong claim in relation to clinical needs.

5

Identity, AIDS and Other Illnesses

In *Safe*, Todd Haynes's 1995 film, a woman's life is disrupted by a mysterious, debilitating illness. The film traces the progressive disintegration of Carol White, employing illness as both literal and metaphorical device, and follows her attempts at reconstruction through a rehabilitation centre working along the lines of Alcoholics Anonymous and other Twelve Step Programmes. What she suffers from is identified as environmental illness, a kind of proliferating allergy in relation to substances in her environment. Potentially nowhere is safe.

As an early contributor to New Queer film-making, Haynes had previously touched on themes linking with AIDS (notably in *Poison* in 1991). Some reviewers were quick to read *Safe* as an AIDS metaphor, perhaps because any illness that really scares will suggest AIDS in the 1990s. But this is to leap to conclusions. Adam Mars-Jones, in his review for the *Independent*, asserted:

> AIDS has a fixed set of cultural meanings, which must either be allowed or contested, while what happens to Carol White (Julianne Moore) is something that she must make sense of as best she can – and so must we – as we watch. (Mars-Jones, 1996)

In Chapter 3 I explored the generation of cultural meanings around AIDS, as exemplified in the work of Susan Sontag, and proposed that such meanings form the context in which individual experiences of HIV and AIDS take shape. Mars-Jones's comment raises the issue of how the subjective experience of different illnesses is influenced by an array of associated cultural meanings, reflecting Sontag's contrasting of AIDS with cancer. One objective of this chapter is to explore comparatively the literature on different forms of chronic illness to see how different meanings underwrite different experiences.

Even if AIDS has a distinctive set of cultural meanings (Mars-Jones overstates the case in saying that it is fixed) the suggestion that this means the person with AIDS has relatively little to make sense of is plainly contradicted by empirical studies. This is one of the limitations in the contributions of some cultural studies academics and other cultural critics to the debates around AIDS: they operate in a world uncluttered by inconvenient or contradictory evidence, and see wider cultural processes as overdetermining individual experience. Similarly, many of the micro-sociological 'experience of illness' studies consider individual life histories in a way that precludes understanding how wider societal processes and discourses impinge on self understanding. A second aim in this chapter is to try to link these two kinds of analysis in exploring the question of how different AIDS is from other forms of chronic illness.

In Chapter 3 the general approach of the sociological 'experience of illness' literature was outlined. Here we will consider the detail of some of these studies to make some empirical comparison with AIDS as a grounded experience, involving the use of health and related services and the relationships that develop between people with AIDS and professionals. Cultural critics and AIDS activists have correctly identified the unique nature of AIDS as a cultural, political and social phenomenon. Yet it is also an illness (or, to be accurate, a syndrome of illnesses) in the body, and there are points of similarity as well as difference with other illnesses.

Multiple sclerosis

In terms of the discussion of stigma and illness, multiple sclerosis (MS) might strike us as self-evidently very different from AIDS. It is a progressively debilitating illness which usually results in an early death, yet it is not caused by a transmissible agent, and it is universally seen as a tragic event (together with, for example, Alzheimer's disease) with the sufferer deserving sympathy and compassion. Think of the ruined career and death of cellist Jacqueline Du Pré. Linked with the sense of tragedy is one of randomness and lack of meaning. Being diagnosed with MS does not associate one with a 'group' having any identifying factor other than the disease. Being diagnosed with HIV often carries associations with socially recognizable stigmatized groups. Ironically, this can have positive effects for the person diagnosed HIV-positive: a gay man is fairly likely to know someone else with HIV or affected by it or working in related fields, and to have access to support through pre-existing social networks. HIV/AIDS is inevitably a dimension of gay self-consciousness in Britain since the mid-1980s. Someone struck down with MS, in contrast, is likely to experience this as a totally individual, unforeseeable and isolating event, which can render coping much more difficult.

If we look instead at the details of daily experience and personal histories with MS, however, we find a number of parallels with the experience of AIDS. In his book on MS Ian Robinson identifies five distinctive features of the disease. Its aetiology is unknown; its onset is variable; diagnosis is problematic; prognosis is unpredictable; and there is no effective treatment. Running throughout these features is the theme of uncertainty, and Robinson asserts that this is a key determinant in the way that sufferers and their social networks respond – that they are pushed towards developing their own strategies for understanding and managing MS (Robinson, 1988, p. 13).

Typically, the onset of symptoms related to MS is very slow. Sufferers tend to put vague, intermittent early symptoms in the explanatory framework of overwork, being 'run down', growing older, and so on, as acceptable explanations for something being 'not quite right' with them. Interestingly, at this stage, before a diagnosis of MS is possible, Robinson reports a 'normative consensus' developing between doctor and patient to view the symptoms as trivial. This may lead to problems later on when a diagnosis of MS is made, since the patient may no longer trust the judgement of the doctor (*ibid.*, p. 21).

The threshold for recognizing symptoms of MS and subsequent actions on the part of the sufferer depend, according to Robinson, on individual social circumstances. In the case of HIV and AIDS, we might argue that this threshold is also closely tied to membership of perceived risk groups for HIV transmission. As with MS, the onset of symptoms associable with HIV can be extremely variable, but the relationship between symptoms and diagnosis is rather different. Furthermore, the causative agent in AIDS is known (or is accepted by most people as known) and its antibodies can be detected using a single, simple test. I described in Chapter 3 a number of circumstances in which people came to have an HIV-antibody test and found themselves to be HIV-positive. For some, it was the result of a search for the explanation of vague, persistent illness, rather as with MS. But this group were a minority. They tended to be the long-term diagnosed at time of interview, or at least those who probably became infected some years before and had gone beyond the so-called latency period of HIV infection: in the mid-1980s the epidemic had not established itself in Britain to any degree and not many people were going for testing speculatively. A greater proportion (more recently diagnosed) perceived that they might be at some risk for HIV through sexual behaviour, injecting drugs use, or being haemophiliac and had, for example, rightly surmised that mild but persistent flu-like illness could be seroconversion. In our research, the greatest number in this category were gay men.[1]

Active resistance to a diagnosis, that is a positive decision not to have an HIV test, was also most associable with gay men, and with a perception they may have been at risk. The rationale here was often 'I'd rather not know, and in any case there isn't a cure.' Other categories of person were more likely to take the test with alacrity, assuming they would be negative.[2]

Perception of personal risk of having acquired HIV (or HIV being an explanation for mysterious illness) was more common among gay men than other categories of our interviewees. But this difference was not solely about autonomous perceptions and decisions around testing. A person presenting to a GP with the vague symptoms associable with HIV infection (and, importantly, a great range of other illnesses) would much more likely be pointed in the direction of an HIV test if identifying as a gay man than as anything else. Willingness to include HIV as a possible diagnosis on the part of the medical professional was influenced by his or her perception of the likely risk profile of the patient: gay men were likely to be regarded as high risk regardless of their actual behaviours.

In sum, though diagnosis and onset of illness have a similarly indeterminate relationship in HIV and MS, the pattern of seeking diagnosis is much more marked in terms of membership of particular groups for HIV than it is for MS. This is clearly linked to HIV being a discreet, transmissible agent, which is generally associated with identifiable risk groups. It would be incorrect to conclude that these differences are absolute, however. We did, for example, interview some gay men who had thought themselves to be at low risk for HIV and whose explanatory frameworks were similar to those of some of Robinson's MS sufferers:

> I just thought, you know, I was getting older, so my body couldn't shake things off so easily. I'd maybe had risky sex once or twice, but that was a long time ago. It was only when I was really ill that time I thought I should have the test.

The progression of the experience of MS following a more or less certain diagnosis is described by Robinson as a complex process which is as much psychosocial as medical. Receipt of diagnosis may be accompanied by shock, anger, grief or fear, but it also commonly results in a sense of relief, in that it acts as a kind of punctuation mark: it means that a label can be attached to symptoms that previously were attended by uncertainty. He draws explicit comparison with diagnosis of epilepsy, which is almost always allied with shock, and sees this as connected with the more stigmatizing nature of epilepsy. Similarly, we have described HIV diagnoses as schismatic, associated both with AIDS being stigmatic and the tendency to see an HIV diagnosis as a death sentence. Here again, though, it is incorrect to draw an absolute comparison. A few of our respondents did report an HIV-positive diagnosis as a relief. These were out gay men who were 'socialized' into the world of HIV in that they knew others who were positive and had maybe also lost friends or partners to AIDS.

> Well, it was all around me anyway. I didn't think there was much chance the result would be negative. And then I thought at least I can commit myself to staying healthy. Not knowing was worse than the possibility of being positive.

The quality of the experience of diagnosis was tied in with the social worlds of individuals.

Autobiographical accounts of life with MS, like those we have described for HIV/AIDS, often focus on living for the present and trying to adopt a healthy lifestyle (Robinson, 1988, p. 40). But indefinite maintenance of health may not be possible in either case, and various analytical concepts have been proposed to describe the social processes associated with worsening health. Goffman's notion of the stigmatized attempting to 'pass' as normal has been modified here in Davis's concept of 'normalization', by which is meant an attempt to carry on life as normal, despite the progressive visibility of illness (Davis, 1963). Even though an illness may not in itself be stigmatizing, the limitations it imposes on full social participation can engender a sense of 'loss of self', of not being a whole person, as discussed in Chapter 3 (see Charmaz, 1983). There is not so much a need to disguise the fact of having the illness absolutely as to mask its debilitating effects. Later on, this masking may no longer be physically possible, and at this point a second explanatory concept becomes relevant, that of 'disassociation' (Cunningham, 1977; Miles, 1979). What is meant here is that the sufferer develops a distinct life based around the illness, with his or her primary reference group becoming others who share the same illness. Disassociation is described as a common pattern in MS by Cunningham, but it is one that is not adopted with alacrity: some of the respondents in Robinson's study did not, for example, want to join MS support groups since this would represent to them a change of identity from the 'community of the healthy' to the 'community of the ill' (Robinson, 1988, p. 116). Some of the people interviewed in the evaluation of the Centre who did not use its services similarly described not wanting to be reminded of their condition by seeing others with HIV/AIDS, and in a study of participants in clinical trials of novel antiviral drugs, Lorna Ryan found 'watching sick people' to be a reason for not wanting to spend more than the minimum necessary time in the clinic (Ryan, 1995, pp. 151–2).

'Passing', 'normalization' and 'disassociation' are all relevant to the discussion of HIV and AIDS, but they exist in a different relation than in a disease that is gradual and incremental. The 'latency' period between HIV infection and AIDS-defining illnesses, often lasting many years, means that 'passing' may be irrelevant, even though HIV and AIDS are stigmatizing. There may be no apparent physical markers, even with an AIDS diagnosis, and it is not uncommon to hear the phrase 'I had no idea he was even ill' when someone suddenly dies from a serious opportunistic infection such as PCP. 'Passing' is relevant, however, where progressive weight loss is a factor or where disfiguring lesions of Kaposi's sarcoma appear on publicly visible parts of the body. So, for example, some AIDS organizations show people how to use make-up to disguise lesions. This said, such physical changes may only occur at a stage of illness where mobility is already quite restricted and not much time is spent in public places or outside the company of the 'own' and the 'wise'.

With HIV and AIDS I would argue that the relationship between 'normalization' and 'disassociation' is far from linear. 'Disassociation' is likely to begin much earlier in the experience of HIV/AIDS than in the case of MS, and this is connected with stigma. On diagnosis, a person with HIV will be made aware of the services that are available, and these include social care organizations which offer a range of practical and social support on their premises.[3] A proportion, as we found in our study, choose to have no contact with services other than regular monitoring of their health status through, for example, hospital GUM clinics. In interviews they described reasons for this such as 'I'm not going to let this take over my life' or 'I just want to carry on as normal'. They would appear to be 'normalizing' their HIV status. Persons in this group were often in full-time employment, and did not want other people's suspicions raised through sudden changes in lifestyle. They tended also to be people from groups who had not been affected by AIDS through their social networks: most of these respondents were heterosexual. As with MS, the capacity to normalize was related to health status, and we found that overall the use of the Centre increased with deteriorating health, at least up to a point where limited mobility made travel to a day centre difficult.

Many others did seek a supportive confidential environment in which to explore how to take their lives forward. We found that use of organizations such as the Centre might begin early after diagnosis, and relatively quickly users began to identify with the Centre as a new 'anchor' in their lives – somewhere in which mutual support was available and where disclosure of HIV status was not threatening. Indeed, several interviewees reported a relief that they could 'be themselves' when at the Centre. In the outside world they did not want their HIV status to be known beyond a very narrow circle (clinical staff, a partner) for fear of persecution. This applied to the asymptomatic as well as the ill, again suggesting the importance of stigma (felt or enacted) in the case of HIV/AIDS.

Gay men tend to constitute the predominant groups and networks within such open-access centres (due in part to the epidemiology of HIV), but other networks develop around targeted services, such as for women or black communities. Over time, involvement in service centres may develop to include volunteering and other forms of active participation, which is allied to the development of a sense of community along various dimensions of identity. These processes have been described in Chapters 3 and 4.

Although the timing and process of 'disassociation' may be rather different for HIV/AIDS, there are parallels with MS in seeking support through non-medical services, and via alternatives to conventional allo-pathic medicine. This similarity appears to lie in the fact that there is no medical cure and both illnesses are marked by progressive deterioration of health, albeit with periods of remission. In the case of MS a number of self-help groups were founded because of the failure of existing services, the recognition of the value of mutual help and the advantages of collective action in lobbying for resources (Robinson, 1988, p. 114–5). Groups such as Body Positive and Frontliners developed along similar lines for HIV/AIDS support, together with organizations promoting treatment activism, including heterodox groups such as Positively Healthy. In the 1980s, first in the United States and later in Britain, the impetus for this came largely from gay activists who perceived govern-mental inertia around an illness seen by the moral majority as the self-inflicted suffering of deviant minorities.

The political and cultural challenges that AIDS posed galvanized a whole movement. For gay men it can be argued that AIDS posed a threat to hard-won senses of identity and community (Kayal, 1993). Such a strong stigma-inspired sense of political expedience never attended MS (or other chronic illnesses; perhaps human-variant CJD is a recent exception), which may explain why the number of MS self-help groups is much smaller. Nonetheless, the organizations in Britain, like AIDS organizations, represent a spectrum of interest from conventional care to activism. Thus, the MS Society offers personal, social and practical help to people with MS, whereas ARMS (Action for Research into MS) tries to influence medical policy and practice out of a concern that not enough is being done.

The various motivations underlying the use of alternative therapies among the HIV-positive was described in Chapter 3. Studies of people with MS indicate some similar rationales for turning to alternative or complementary therapies, which reflect the lack of a cure and the prob-lematic nature of doctor–patient relationships. Especially when illness worsens, the lack of effectiveness of allopathic treatments can bring about a willingness to try whatever else is available. Other reasons reported in studies of MS patients included concern over wasting doctors' time, poor experience of previous medical contacts and the relatively easy access to and unhurried appointments available with alternative practitioners (Robinson, 1988, p. 87). This might be labelled opportunistic or pragmatic use of such therapies. Additionally, there are some people who turn to such therapies explicitly as part of a philosophy of developing an holistic approach to health.

Doctor–patient relations

The 'experience of illness' literature places strong emphasis on the role of doctor–patient relationships in chronic illness. It highlights how the development of such relationships influences the decisions that the patient makes about treatment, as well as the doctor. Chronicity both prolongs the relationship and changes its quality, when compared with acute illness. The key element is that in the absence of a cure the doctor is not regarded as an omniscient being, and a crisis of confidence may result. With MS, a kind of eclecticism is common, in which patients use formal advice from doctors as only one element in reaching decisions about their health care and lives more generally. This is also the case with HIV/AIDS. In both cases new therapies (both conventional and alternative) become available from time to time, but there is a significant difference in perspective on their use between doctor and patient. What the doctors' perspective fails to take into account, according to Robinson, is that patients always self-manage illness to some extent; that aside from the strictures of medical ethics, people will try whatever treatments become available where there are no proven therapies; and, perhaps most importantly, that from the patients' perspective what matters is the illness in the context of their overall lives, and that a sense of control over life is maintained (*ibid.*, p. 91).

This sense of control is related by Robinson to a struggle over defining the boundaries of MS, and who can legitimately decide these boundaries. If an individual can define what the experience of MS means, then a greater sense of control may be achievable. With time, the explanatory framework of conventional medicine may seem progressively less adequate, and a sense may grow that the doctors' opinions can be legitimately challenged. We saw in Chapter 3 how an individual reacted to the sense of loss of control and being used as a guinea-pig. He thought that the pursuit of a number of invasive tests by the doctors had more to do with their curiosity in investigating HIV than that they were likely to be able to do anything to improve his condition. 'It's my body after all', as he put it. So the theme of control of knowledge around HIV echoes research on MS. What is different is that the narratives surrounding clinical professional–patient relationships tended to be elaborated in identity terms where HIV was concerned, that is for those with negatively marked identities, such as gay men and injecting drugs users. For example, one man here discusses his experience of a home support nursing team:

> I got home and tried to manage on my own. I ended up going back to [the hospital] and seeing P. And I said I just can't manage. I said, I wasn't even asked on the ward if I wanted any help when I went home. . . . And so he got people to come in and do the shopping, meals on wheels and so on. And again it was all, how can I put it? Very anti-gay. S was the only one who was helpful, and I presume he was gay, but I don't know. He was so nice. But there were two staff nurses, one in particular, who was totally anti-gay, totally, didn't want anything to do with HIV infection.

Notice the conflation in the last sentence of HIV status and being gay. Many gay respondents emphasized the homophobic reactions of nursing and medical staff (especially in the 1980s). Some knowledge and attitude studies of professionals coincide with these reports, in that they revealed negative moral judgements on gay men (see Feldman, Garside and Gatter, 1996, for various examples). In the period since our research was undertaken, knowledge and attitudes in relation to gay men seem gradually to have improved, with the progressive professionalization of HIV/AIDS services. Problems remain, though. A recent study concerning the transfer of HIV/AIDS care to Primary Health Care Teams (as part of the move to Care in the Community) still found homophobic attitudes among some doctors (Winn, 1997).

Other chronic illnesses

Based on the example of MS, we have traced how the 'experience of illness' literature illuminates chronic illness in a sociological sense by reference to identifiable stages of illness, attendant social effects and derived analytical concepts. Onset and diagnosis, progression, psychosocial adjustment, the development of significant relationships (including with the medical profession), exploration of self-help groups and a turn to non-conventional therapies are themes as relevant to HIV/AIDS as they are to MS, though we have begun to indicate that the experience of HIV/AIDS tends to be influenced by identity factors more significantly than is MS.

A significant difference between MS and HIV/AIDS is the potential for HIV/AIDS to be stigmatizing. It is relevant, then, to make some further comparisons with chronic illnesses that do involve stigma.

Alongside cancer, whose stigmatizing capacity was outlined by Susan Sontag (1991), perhaps the classic example of a stigmatizing chronic condition, at least as regarded by the literature, is epilepsy. Like many other chronic illnesses, the underlying causes of epilepsy are poorly understood, its onset may be gradual, its diagnosis ambiguous, and its prognosis unpredictable. With the advent of drug treatments it is less likely to lead to fatalities than in the past, and indeed treatment can in some cases be curative.

In his careful analysis of epilepsy, Scambler (1989) argues that the fear and associated stigma are perhaps overstated now, though they remain very real for the epileptic. A negative stereotype is conventionally accepted as having arisen from the classic, and stereotypical, presentation of the illness: the *grand mal* seizure. An apparently normal person will, a propos no visible cause, enter a fit in which there is no voluntary control of the body, and indeed the body may undergo violent and distressing muscular spasms. This at least is the supposed stereotype. And associated with the public display of a disturbing loss of bodily control, a set of intractable popular ideas is thought to remain about the meaning of these seizures: that they indicate an underlying mental disorder, and, connected with this, that epilepsy is associable with anti-social personality traits (Scambler, 1989, p. 41).

In fact, several empirical studies of public attitudes to epilepsy reveal them to be far less negative than they were in the past, and that there is now a degree of public sympathy for the condition, at least in Britain (*ibid.*). But historically epilepsy has been so powerfully stigmatizing that even now receipt of a diagnosis characteristically induces strong fears of stigmatization:

most people are extremely upset when first learning of the diagnosis of epilepsy. This is fundamentally because they see epilepsy
as stigmatizing, a perception rooted in their partial and idiosyncratic internalizations of lay beliefs, attitudes, and practices
concerning people with epilepsy. (*ibid.*, p. 75)

The divergence between independently assessed public knowledge and
attitudes, and private perceptions among the epileptic, leads Scambler to
make a distinction between perceived versus experienced stigma (the two
often are not consonant). This is to repeat, in a slightly different form,
Goffman's separation of felt stigma from enacted stigma. As in discussions of other stigmatizing chronic illnesses, it is argued for epilepsy that
felt stigma is often more significant and debilitating than enacted stigma.
The question of the extent to which felt stigma is justified has not been
answered: a general survey of public attitudes cannot map directly onto
the lived experiences of individual epileptics. What Scambler does instead
is to analyse the mechanisms through which the separation of perceived
from experienced stigma arises for epilepsy, and how it is sustained.

The key lies in social networks and the process of socialization. For
epilepsy, the family is the crucible in which self-perception as an epileptic
takes place. This may seem trivial, since the family (whatever form it may
take) is formative for self-perception along many dimensions, but epilepsy as a phenomenon with an associated set of lay beliefs has a specific
relation with family and socialization. Within the family, the epileptic
individual learns to fear enacted stigma. The classic response to this fear
is to try, as far as possible, to avoid disclosure of epileptic status to others
outside the family, in other words to 'pass' as normal. In some cases
concealment may even be within the family (*ibid.*, p. 82). In epilepsy the
family often reinforces the message that epilepsy is shameful and best
kept hidden. It is directly implicated in the growth of a life based on
strategies to avoid enacted stigma (what Scambler terms the *hidden
distress* model). On one hand this is about protecting the family member
from discrimination. It is often the case that the parents and spouses of
epileptics are over-protective, and this can lead to dependency. Just as
importantly, however, a key lay belief about epilepsy is that it is heredi-
tary, that it runs in families. Coupled with the idea that epilepsy is at the
least an imperfection, this often leads to a sort of collective family shame
around the epileptic. The fact of epilepsy is believed to be a reflection on

the family as a whole. For example, in one study a parent of an epileptic was quoted as saying:

> People shy away, and they immediately think there's something wrong with the rest of the family because you've got one like that. (West, 1986, p. 255)

Families may therefore share and be instrumental in inculcating stigma and blame in the epileptic.

We have already argued that HIV and AIDS are stigmatizing. Concealment of HIV status (or perhaps, more accurately, non-disclosure) is common, especially in the time immediately following diagnosis. But in what senses are stigma and associated non-disclosure the same phenomena in epilepsy and HIV/AIDS? We need to consider both the cultural construction of stigma and what kind of epileptic or person living with HIV/AIDS we are imagining. Scambler argues that with shifts in the public perception of epilepsy, it is now best characterized as an *ontological deficit*, that is an imperfection of being for which the sufferer bears no moral responsibility (Scambler, 1989, p. 49). To be epileptic is to be unlucky. HIV and AIDS are different in that there is a popular cultural association between 'deviant subcultures' and the virus. There are still many conservative people who see those living with HIV and AIDS as being morally culpable for their serostatus.

Interviewing users of an AIDS service organization about their life histories since diagnosis elicited many harrowing tales of enacted stigma.

> I've been stabbed several times. The second time was in the middle of the afternoon, in the flats where I live, on the corridor. He shouted some anti-gay AIDS abuse and then stabbed me. And then he went out and slashed a man's face. But what got me was the police actually told the other victim that I was HIV-positive. I don't know whether it was his relatives or his sons and that, but after this happened I started getting excreta through the door, pushed through the letterbox. ... And it got to the stage I was so frightened, if I heard voices in the corridor and I was about to go out, I would wait until those voices disappeared before I even attempted to go out. (Gay man in his forties)

Two points about the person are salient to the argument here. First, he was an openly gay man adopting the dress and personal style of an easily recognizable gay urbanite. Secondly, he was living alone on an inner-city council estate. He had received threats and abuse from youths living on the estate who had assumed he 'had AIDS' because they thought he was gay. As he suffered further illness and lost weight, they seemed confirmed in their assumption. For this interviewee and for other gay men and IDUs fear of enacted stigma was soundly related to experienced consequences of disclosure (or assumptions made by others about HIV status). It was more realistic perhaps than in the case of epilepsy.

Other kinds of people in our study had experienced adverse reactions when their positive status was suspected, or known, by others.

> I was living with my brother. And he wasn't around much because of working in [country outside Europe]. His wife is always here. She was all right at first, but when I got ill and started going to the clinic she started suspecting that I was HIV-positive because of where we come from, and she started mistreating me. She stopped me from using the washing machine and things like that. She has sisters here, but they don't even want to stop and say hello to me, because they are afraid of being seen with me. (East African woman in her thirties, partner of a political refugee who had since died)

Such experiences, nevertheless, were qualitatively different from those of gay men. Interviewees who were heterosexual and with no injecting drugs use history may have feared disclosure, but tended to find that strangers and workers in public service settings did not expect HIV to be among their problems. Again, it was the association of HIV with particular identities that was significant. Among heterosexual interviewees there were some, however, who were particularly fearful about disclosure of status to their social networks. These were East African women, such as the person quoted above. For them factors to do with their cultural identities and attitudes to AIDS underpinned the fear of enacted stigma. In this case, the stigma had been enacted: the grounds for fear were real. African immigrants face acute problems of ostracism and discrimination in their communities of origin.

These kinds of discrimination based on irrational fears of contamination and allied forms of prejudice such as homophobia are quite different from the stigma attaching to epilepsy. In both cases there are additional forms of discrimination which are best conceived separately since they may have some basis in rationality. Epileptics, if known to be such, are banned from holding a driving licence or operating heavy machinery in the workplace. Sound arguments defending these restrictions can be put forward in terms of the safety of the epileptic and other road users or workers. In the case of HIV, insurance companies, especially where life assurance is concerned, may not offer cover or will refuse to pay out on claims where the individual is known to be HIV-positive. Though this may not seem politically acceptable, it is rational within the terms of what an insurance company exists to do: make money by offering cover while accepting what on balance are relatively good risks. A person who is HIV-positive statistically (at least until very recently) has a much greater chance of dying prematurely than someone who is not, all else being equal. What is less justifiable is for an insurance company to refuse cover or load a premium because the individual is known or assumed to be a gay man. Here, an assumption is made that being gay equates with a quantifiable risk of being or becoming HIV-positive. The argument is unsustainable, and prejudicial. Similarly, in the workplace a person may be refused a job or forced out because of HIV status. There may be some rational basis for this in terms of employing someone who will not be able to carry out their job properly; but equally management might feel that an HIV-positive employee may have an adverse influence in the working environment, or even place colleagues at risk of acquiring the virus. The latter is likely to be pure fantasy.

Legitimate discrimination in the public sphere where epilepsy is concerned would seem to be fairly clear-cut, whereas it is much more ambiguous for HIV. This difference is another reflection of the moral prejudice attending HIV stigma, coupled to the real difference that HIV can be transmitted between individuals whereas epilepsy cannot (except genetically). Even then, fears around HIV transmission are often unrealistic and confused with fears about homosexuality. The likelihood of experiencing these forms of discrimination again relates to the kind of individual involved. Middle-class gay men working in the care professions are likely to have better protection of their employment and work in an environment where colleagues are well informed about HIV and anti-discrimination policies are in place than, say, someone working on a building site.

> I've had to be off work since Christmas. I've remained in regular contact to know what's going on. Some months ago D came up with a proposal which amounts to me being very much a free agent, so I can work from home with all the necessary office facilities. They've put an enormous amount of trust in me, and I'm very grateful for that. (Gay man in his fifties, in a senior position in Social Services)

Those who are more privileged according to general social indicators are less exposed to enacted stigma surrounding HIV/AIDS than the less privileged. Aside from working environment, they are likely to be owner-occupiers and therefore less exposed to the kinds of social stress typifying life on inner-city housing estates. This is perhaps a general feature of living with chronic illnesses in which HIV and AIDS are not so different from other conditions. Based on employment statistics, Scambler argues that working-class people are particularly vulnerable to unemployment because of epilepsy: 75 per cent of those unemployed in his sample were working-class (Scambler, 1989, p. 95). Relative social and economic status influence experience of illness across a broad spectrum of problems.

Disclosure of HIV status within the private sphere, that is the networks of a person's family, partners, intimates and friends, seems rather different from disclosure of epilepsy. Most of our interviewees were gay men whose social circumstances differed significantly from Scambler's study sample. They had been infected with HIV as adults, at which time they were not living with their immediate biological family, and, given the tendency of gay men to migrate to major urban centres (Johnson *et al.*, 1994; Kelley, Pebody and Scott, 1996; Cant, 1997), often at some distance from them. The issue of disclosure of HIV status was in several cases confounded with the fact that the men had not come out to their families. They felt they faced the double trauma of declaring their sexual orientation as well as a stigmatizing illness simultaneously. Some had done this, whereas others felt the experience would be too distressing to their families. In contrast, where disclosure to circles of friends on the gay scene was concerned, about half of the gay interviewees felt that it was safe and even advantageous, since it could enable peer support. The rest did not see the gay scene as a supportive environment and feared ostracism and sexual rejection if they were 'public' about their status, and in other research we found that some gay scene venues came to have reputations for having HIV-positive customers, which could deter HIV-positive men from going there (Annetts, Eisenstadt and Gatter, 1996, p. 41).

Where sexual partners were concerned, there are similarities between HIV/AIDS and epilepsy in that it is usual to disclose only to long-term partners. The underlying reasons for this seem, however, to diverge. In epilepsy, the risk of inadvertent disclosure in casual sexual encounters (via a fit) is relatively low and announcing epilepsy in advance might be assumed to invite rejection (another example of felt stigma). In long-term relationships with an intimate partner concealment would be practically impossible. With HIV, initial concealment is possible. Among our interviewees the majority concealed HIV status from casual partners, explaining that they always practised safer sex in this context and that disclosure to a stranger carried risks of malicious exposure. The others told all potential sexual partners, even at the risk of rejection, out of fear of infecting someone else, no matter how small the risk of the sexual contact.

In long-term relationships, disclosure became practically unavoidable. A desire to practise unprotected anal intercourse in a stable intimate relationship was common, and this inevitably raised the issue of negotiated safety and the possible infection of a negative partner. Even if this was not a factor, at some point chronic illness would almost inevitably raise the question of HIV in a relationship.

For other people, the possibilities of concealment were linked with whether they belonged to populations thought of as being at risk. Here, East African women (even more so than their partners) were in a doubly difficult situation. Especially if from Uganda, with one of the most devastating AIDS epidemics in the world, there was a strong possibility for them that 'mysterious' illnesses would be attributed by others to HIV. But at the same time, as we have seen, the shame and ostracism that can attach to being HIV-positive in East African communities means there may be a strong desire to conceal a positive status, even from a partner. Indeed, several of the women we spoke to reported finding out, in this country, that they were HIV-positive only after their partners had died with AIDS. Injecting drugs users also found their worlds infected with the suspicion of HIV: HIV is part of the argot of drugs-using subcultures, revealed to a wider public, for example, in Irvine Welsh's novels, particularly *Trainspotting*.

Again, those without marked minority identities generally found the possibilities for concealment of HIV status greater, both within their own social networks and communities and outside them. For example, one heterosexual woman met her partner while holidaying in a sub-Saharan African country. They planned to marry and for him to come over to England. In the meantime he became ill and died. The woman, who was white and middle-class, tested positive for HIV. She was also working in a profession involving contact with children, which meant she felt very strongly that her status must not become public as it could well lose her her job. She felt confident that she could keep her status concealed, as she continued in good health and there was no reason for anyone to make an association between her and HIV. Her visits to the GUM clinic for monitoring could simply be explained away as 'appointments'.

> I think in the beginning it was difficult because of a fear of being found out. I had this big secret about myself that I didn't want other people to know. So that was hard. But as time goes on it just gets easier. It's just part of me, it's a part of me that other people don't need to know. I just carry on as normal. ... Because of working with children, confidentiality was a big worry. But I think public opinion is becoming more sensitive and I'm less worried and also I realize the chance of it being found out is unlikely as well.

Gender

The discussion of identity so far in this chapter has centred on the degree of cultural association made between identities and HIV/AIDS. As even a cursory glance at cultural debates will show, a further key identity factor central to societal discourse, in Britain and elsewhere, is gender. Continuing a comparison between HIV/AIDS and other forms of chronic illness, I turn now to consider illnesses in which gender inevitably plays a role, specifically illnesses that affect women exclusively, or almost exclusively. To what extent is gender itself a central explanatory factor in the way these illnesses are experienced and gain social currency? And does HIV/ AIDS engage with gender in comparable ways?

The two examples I will consider are breast cancer[4] and menstrual disorders, illnesses featured in the Routledge 'Experience of Illness' series. In discussing breast cancer, Fallowfield and Clark (1991) find features of women's experience of diagnosis and treatment that closely parallel the examples discussed earlier. Stigma plays a role, in that some people fear contagion from someone with cancer, regardless of type (Verres, 1986). There is also a tendency, similar to that described by Susan Sontag, for some women to blame themselves for getting breast cancer, as if it were divine retribution for 'immoral' behaviours or an otherwise unhealthy lifestyle:

> When I found the lump I knew exactly what it was and I thought this is punishment at last for what I did. You see I had an illegitimate baby when I was 19 and I kept her. (Quotation from interviewee in Fallowfield and Clark, 1991, p. 22)

Unlike this respondent, Fallowfield and Clark found that many of the women in their study went through an initial period of denial on finding a breast lump. Such denial is similar to that found in many other chronic illnesses, including HIV/AIDS. Subsequent psychological adjustment also shows a common pattern with other illnesses: a mixture of fighting spirit and stoic acceptance on the one hand; anxiety, depression and a sense of hopelessness on the other.

Breast cancer is of course not necessarily fatal, but the long-term success of treatment cannot be assured. As with other cancers, the location and size of tumours, and whether they have metastasized,[5] are critical factors. The experience of cancers can therefore be divided into pre- and post-operative phases (where treatment is possible and accepted by the sufferer). Post-operatively and during radiotherapy or chemo-therapy the cancer patient is likely to come into contact with those who are dying, and it is common at this stage for any persistent denial to end. Beyond this point there may be further anxiety and depression, physical and sexual dysfunction, and social withdrawal (depending on the post-treatment prognosis). On the other hand, the cancer can become a positive focus around which life values are adjusted (*ibid.*, p. 73). Identification with and participation in cancer support groups are often part of this process of readjusting to 'living with cancer'. For others, support groups are not appealing either because of practical problems in attending them, or because of fears of seeing very ill people, wishing to forget cancer in everyday life, and not liking participation in group discussions (*ibid.*, p. 112).

These kinds of processes connected with adjusting to life with a life-threatening illness very closely parallel our findings with people living with HIV and AIDS. With a chance that breast cancer is incurable via conventional medicine, there is also an equivalent interest in the use of alternative and complementary therapies. In the British context the best-known example of this is the Bristol Cancer Help Centre, which offers combined therapy based on diet, megavitamins and psychological input. As in our research, there is also a tendency in advanced cancer for patients either to strike out on their own, feeling that the medical profession can do no more for them, or alternatively to take a dependent position in relation to conventional medical wisdom, even though it provides no universal solutions (*ibid.*, pp. 115–16).

Fallowfield and Clark wrote their book from the perspective of authors trained in the medical field (one a nurse, the other a consultant surgeon). This is not insignificant, since it creates a rather different emphasis from other books in the same series written by sociologists. In examining lay attitudes and beliefs about cancer, the response to discovering a breast lump and diagnosis, the psychosocial outcome of treatment and subsequent psychological reactions to recurrence, it is clear that the evidence is being reviewed from a biomedically informed position. So, for example, lay attitudes and beliefs are reviewed from the perspective of their rationality; and where found to be irrational they are explained as having a psychological function in terms of giving meaning to illness. There is implicit always the assertion of medical 'truths':

> This [poor understanding of the etiology and biology of cancer] can make it difficult at times to challenge some of the popular myths and fears that lay people can often harbour about causal factors, prevalence of the disease, and its curability relative to other life-threatening illnesses. However, an appreciation of some of these lay attitudes and beliefs about breast cancer has important implications for the utilization of screening services and the psychological aspects of patient care. (*ibid.*, p. 17)

Given the high degree of public attention given to breast cancer now, for example the pink ribbon campaign, echoing the red ribbon campaign for AIDS, and the fact that breast cancer affects one in fourteen women in Britain, Fallowfield and Clark's book is peculiarly silent on the issue of gender, where a more sociological perspective might see it as a central factor. Attention is given to the psychological impact of mastectomy, especially the effects on body image and associated sexual dysfunction. But there is no attempt to locate the psychological dimension within cultural values concerning what it is to be a man or a woman, or what masculinity and femininity mean. There is some brief discussion of male partners' reactions to women's surgery (*ibid.*, p. 71) but no wider consideration of how men's views of women influence the subjective experience of breast cancer for women. A gendered perspective is also absent where self-blame for acquiring cancer is concerned:

> This is God's punishment for my wickedness. I had an affair once with a married man. I'd always had large breasts and that's what attracted him I suppose. (*ibid.*, p. 22)

In our research we found some gay men who saw their infection with HIV as a consequence of a reckless lifestyle. In his final article for the *Guardian* (published posthumously) Oscar Moore, author of the paper's regular PWA column, expressed such a view:

> The heights may have left us giddy, but we were having too much fun to want to come down. And yet come down we would. We had been partying so hard that the hangover had to be harder. (Moore, *Guardian Weekend*, 21 September 1996)

But there is a quality in this kind of rationalization for AIDS that is different from that expressed by the woman for her breast cancer. Even if gay men blame themselves in some way for having HIV, it is on the basis of a shared culpability derived from what in a sense is collective pleasure. This is different from the account of the woman, since it implies self-blame conditioned by a subordinate gender position. Her sexuality had tempted a man, and this immorality rebounded to her disadvantage. Oscar Moore and the gay men we interviewed may have felt a moral dimension to self-blame, but this was in terms of physical excess rather than any sin-like manipulation of others through gendered attributes.

Annette and Graham Scambler's (1993) book about menstrual disorders strikes a contrast with Fallowfield and Clark, since they frame their discussion from the outset with a discussion of gender, as do writers commenting from perspectives other than medicine or medical sociology, a good example being Sophie Law's *Issues of Blood* (1990) which contextualizes clinical aspects of menstruation within a feminist political analysis of the phenomenon. The Scamblers explore the significance of the fact that medicine has historically been a male-dominated profession, and how this influences the interplay between medical practice and illnesses which are gender specific. In the nineteenth century popular cultural constructions of the nature of man and woman became written into the thinking of medicine. Foucault documents this well in the first volume of *The History of Sexuality* (1978). The process was perhaps most insidious in the nascent discipline of psychiatry, where the emotions and personalities of women were seen to be irrational (at least compared to men's) and under the direct control of their reproductive systems: the term *hysteria* comes directly from the ancient Greek for womb (*hysteros*).

Concerning menstrual disorders specifically, the Scamblers discuss how menstruation came to be seen as a pathological process during the nineteenth century:

> It yet evidently lies on the borders of pathological change, as it is evidenced not only by the pain which so frequently accompanies it and the local and constitutional disorders which so frequently arise in this connection, but by the general systemic disturbance and local histological changes of which the discharge is merely the outward expression and result. (Geddes and Thompson, 1890. Quoted in Scambler and Scambler, 1993, p. 22)

Such influence is still felt today in the way that medical practitioners treat menstrual disorders, and in the perceptions that women themselves have of menstruation. The Scamblers review studies of women's perceptions of menstruation and find that beliefs, usually acquired at an early age, reflect general cultural stereotypes of menstruation as being a negative and symptom-laden phenomenon (Scambler and Scambler, 1993, p. 30). In their own studies they found that women often considered 'normal' menstruation cycles to be akin to illness, or at least inconvenient. Disturbances to menstruation, such as amenorrhoea, menorrhagia and dysmenorrhoea may then be constructed by women as simply an extension of something that is already hedged around with taboo and social and physical discomfort. Their decisions to seek or not seek help, and whether informally or through the medical profession, are influenced by such views. The construction of menstruation as a 'woman's problem' tends to mean that women initially seek help through informal networks when they perceive abnormality in their cycles. These networks include partners (whether male or female, though Scambler and Scambler only discuss husbands) and almost exclusively female networks of family and friends (*ibid.*, p. 48).

Scambler and Scambler emphasize that both historical and anthropological sources record that menstruation has taboos associated with it in almost all human societies. Menstrual blood is very often viewed as a source of female power, and inimical to the interests of men. Menstruation, menstrual blood and semen are central to the symbolic construction of gender in many societies (Brandes, 1981; Herdt, 1983; McCormack, 1982; Shuttle and Redgrove, 1980). It is therefore unsurprising that gender becomes an inescapable dimension in the discussion of menstrual disorders, at least from a sociological perspective. But if there is a general problem of a gender-biased medicalization of women's bodies by an inherently patriarchal medical profession, gender must form an important component in the understanding of any illness or disease. What is there to say about HIV and AIDS in terms of gender?

With a steady growth in the numbers of HIV-infected women in Europe and North America, organizations specific to women have multiplied, together with women-specific services in many ASOs. In Britain, for example, there are Positively Women and the Body Positive Women's Group. Service organizations such as the Centre run women-only evenings. Analyses of the emergence of HIV/AIDS as an issue for women have come in parallel, both from academics and those involved in campaigning and service provision.

In terms of generating an overview of HIV and AIDS as gendered phenomena, Cindy Patton's work in the United States is influential. Decoding the political and cultural context in which HIV and AIDS affect women has been central to Patton's project as cultural activist and analyst. The professionalization and 'putting into discourse' of AIDS were at the heart of *Inventing AIDS* (Patton, 1990), themes extended to thinking specifically about women in *Last Served? Gendering the HIV Pandemic* (Patton, 1994). In this latter work she is concerned with looking at women's experience of HIV/AIDS in the wider context of how gender disadvantage affects their health. As in *Inventing AIDS*, she examines how the discourses of AIDS both exclude women, and include them in inappropriate ways. She stresses the need to avoid conceiving women as a homogeneous group with common identities (a characteristic failing of paternalistic discourses) and points up how epidemiology and health promotion misrepresent and fail four kinds of woman. Specifically, she sees categories of identity and community used inappropriately as devices for conceptualizing women's needs in relation to HIV/AIDS as follows:

1. The use of 'heterosexual woman' as an epidemiological category most often implies a notion of risk attaching to a male partner, and subordination to that partner. Patton insists that women do not live in a community defined by their relationship to men.
2. Sex workers to some degree may be described as a community, since they often can be identified in spatial and cultural terms as belonging to oppositional communities. However, in the thinking of public health they tend to be constructed as a risk group for men, not vice versa. This is connected with the stigmatization of sex work. Furthermore, the notion of sex work is ethnocentric, since activities we might label 'prostitution' may have very different meanings in non-Western contexts.
3. The female partners of haemophiliac men are treated as if they form a category, but they don't have any shared, marked identity.
4. Finally, lesbians are in the difficult position of being a community of identity at variance with epidemiological perceptions of risk. (Patton, 1994, Chapter 3)

In similar vein, Robin Gorna, writing in Britain, highlights the tendency for the media to infantilize or demonize women and their sexuality, while also 'heterosexualizing' women's experience of AIDS (by which she means treating women as subordinate to a male partner). In relation to HIV, Gorna sees women as being characterized as vessels and vectors, that is that they are repositories of the virus and responsible for passing it to men. In other words, the kinds of stereotypes of women's sexuality that are rehearsed in a patriarchal society get reinforced by HIV/AIDS. As with gay men, an illness that links sexuality with death is fertile ground for the scapegoating of subordinated sexual identities (Gorna, 1996).

Both writers are describing the formation of discourses around women and AIDS within the medical and allied professions. These affect both the way women are treated by 'the system' and how they understand their own experience of HIV and AIDS. In interviewing women about their experiences of living with HIV, we found that several of the themes highlighted by Patton and Gorna were prominent. A clear distinction can be made, however, between experiences that are clearly gendered but not articulated as such, and those where women explicitly linked what had happened to them with the fact that they were women. Indeed, some women didn't discuss living with HIV in gendered terms at all, whereas others clearly framed their own and others' experiences as being peculiar to women. I suggest that these differences are linked to the wider identifications of the women involved; or, to express this another way, that they vary with the women's differing subject positions.

Experiences surrounding childbirth and the raising of children featured strongly as a gendered experience. Yet these were also the experiences that tended not to be articulated from an explicitly gendered position. Particularly in the 1980s, perinatal experiences of HIV-positive women in hospital could be very distressing. The following is an extended extract from one woman's narrative, which illustrates well the point made by Gorna that women's needs may be treated by health professionals as residual to those of their children:

> In the beginning of 19 . . . , I was pregnant, and my husband was ill, and he was tested as one of the first tests they did to try and find out what was wrong with him. And when it came through as being positive, I was six months pregnant. And they said we have to test because you're pregnant.
>
> I was immediately referred to the obstetrician who said I would like you to come and meet the paediatrician. And the paediatrician went away and looked up a lot of paperwork and said I'm very sorry your baby will have not more than a fifty-fifty chance of being, still being alive at two years old. And she'll be born well, it

will be born well, but if you were any less pregnant we would recommend abortion.

When G was born it was just an awful experience. The way I was treated in hospital was just awful. She was three weeks early and both consultants were taking a last-minute holiday before all hell broke loose at the hospital with me. Because they hadn't told anyone. They decided to keep it under their hat because they knew it was going to be very difficult. And they all panicked and there was nobody there who knew me or could support me.

Everyone was too frightened to come near me. And then after G was born she was taken away to the intensive care unit. They wouldn't give her to me to hold. They gave her to my husband to hold. They wouldn't give her to me . . . They wouldn't let me go on to the ward, which they told me I would be after the delivery, I would be just treated as a normal person. I wasn't. I was put in a broom cupboard basically. They had a big cupboard that they'd put a bed in and they put some paper towels on it, and nobody came near me there. Nobody was allowed to see me. The nursing staff didn't come and see me. It was just awful. And nobody came and told me whether my baby was all right.

Later experiences connected with children focused on fears over care for the child should the mother fall ill or die, and concerns over possible breaches of confidentiality, referring either to the child learning inadvertently of the mother's status, or repeating that knowledge to others. Most of the women we interviewed who had children were lone parents, heightening their concerns in these two areas:

When you have children you come into contact with an awful lot of people. Some you know well, some you don't. But you come into contact with lots of people from all sorts of areas. And yeah, that made me feel just very very uneasy. And I didn't go to any more women's groups after that.

What worries me is me getting sick and who will look after J. Even if I had to go into hospital just for a week, who would look after him? He would be so distressed at me having to go into hospital. He would be taken away from his home and be staying with different people that he likes but ... he's not that fond of any particular person.

A mother working in an AIDS support organization:

He's eight. Sometimes he's been here and I've been talking and I'd forget that he was behind me and he's heard me say 'Oh, yes, because I'm positive' or something. And then he'd say to me 'Oh, you're positive, aren't you?' and I just lied. I said 'No, no, no. You got it all wrong.' I think that at the back of his mind he might know a little bit.

It emerged that children's ages had direct practical consequences in terms of the use of AIDS service organizations. As soon as they began to learn to read, and to hear about and ask questions concerning HIV and AIDS, their mothers had to reconsider visiting centres with them, and what alternative childcare arrangements could be made, if at all. There was in a sense a transitional period from about the age of seven to adolescence (though a variable one) where the problems surrounding non-disclosure of HIV status to children were particularly acute. Beyond a certain age mothers felt it would be practically impossible to maintain secrecy, and that in any case a time would come where the child might become able to deal with the practical and emotional implications of their mother's (and possibly their own) positive serostatus.

Among African immigrant women the problems relating to children were likely to be more acute than for our other interviewees. Being here often as refugees, seeking political asylum, meant that families had become divided. Ugandan women discussed how their major concern was getting their children over to Britain, and how difficult this was until they had been granted refugee status by the Home Office.

The role of carer, as Gorna suggests, featured largely in the lives of our women interviewees, a role that tended to extend beyond childcare. As key supporters in their networks of family and friends, they sometimes suppressed their own needs in order to serve others:

I'm basically very healthy. I mean I keep getting a bit thin but I think a lot of that was pressure, stress, and having to be all things to everyone. (Woman, in her thirties, with a young child)

The women who articulated their experiences explicitly in terms of being women were generally those who were not mothers. Possibly this is connected with women being socialized into subordinating their own needs to those of their children. Women without children engaged with HIV/AIDS services as adult individuals and with more time to reflect on their own needs and interests. Using one-to-one services such as counselling, financial advice and alternative therapies was not problematic. It was in the setting of support groups and general drop-in facilities that these women expressed some reservations. These focused on what might be described as gendered social worlds. Because of the history of the way in which such groups were set up, at the time of our research (early 1990s) many of the available groups consisted predominantly of gay men (with the notable exception of those run by Positively Women). In these settings our interviewees often felt that they were in a minority where their particular needs as women were marginalized, if not ignored altogether. One woman, an ex-drug user, had found a Twelve Step Programme for the HIV-positive in which she felt alienated:

> I attended this group for a year and except for one week I have always been the only woman there. And it's quite hard you know. I mean in a way I don't particularly mind and I feel quite comfortable with gay men. I go to Body Positive a lot and I'm usually one of the very few women or the only woman. In the AA group we talk about feelings and what's happening in our lives, and I've got to know the men and they've got to know me. And I do feel very well accepted in that. But it's a bit isolating when time and again you're the only woman there and they quite often discuss their sort of, I don't know, things that aren't relevant to me you know, like the sexual side of their life, cruising, you know, or cottaging. It doesn't mean anything to me and I know it's part of their lives and they have every right to talk about it there.

When she began to use a women-only support group run by Positively Women a whole area of support opened up:

> It's just a difference, right, to see women and children instead of gay men, you know. And I think it's easier to talk. It is, I think. 'Cause there are totally different issues that surround women

really, especially if you've got children, though I haven't. I remember four years ago I did offer to do some voluntary work at ... I definitely got the vibe that you know because I was a woman and drug user, that they didn't really want to know, it really was a sort of gay men's club. I remember being really upset over that because I mean we're talking about a life-threatening illness you know, which has got to go far beyond sexuality.

Out of her concerns for the downplaying of women's needs and interests, this woman had gone on to voluntary and later paid work in services specifically for women. At other points in her interview she raised other concerns specific to women, such as the importance of regular gynaecological checks. She was also at pains to speak up for women who would find gay culture more alien than herself, and for whom a sexualized environment was inappropriate (for example non-British women and mothers bringing their children to HIV/AIDS service centres).

Unlike some of the heterosexual men we interviewed, none of the women expressed open dislike of gay men associable with homophobia. The sense we were given, as in the quotation above, was that the sexualized discourse of gay men in groups was something most women felt uninterested in. In Ryan's study of clinical trial participants she likewise found that the 'sexualization' of the clinic by gay men had a profound influence on how the place was experienced (Ryan, 1995, p. 155). Many of our gay male interviewees, by the same token, were not interested in discussing parenting, or being around children (though these two forms of difference were not equally marked for all women and all gay men).

HIV-positive women who became actively involved in HIV/AIDS organizations, such as the woman described above, found that their experiences as users of organizations shaped their desire to work for women in such settings. Indeed, considering the wider context of women's HIV/AIDS organizations in Britain, it is the case that several of them, including Positively Women, were set up precisely because women using the generic or gay organizations found that their specific needs were not being met.

Through involvement particularly in Positively Women, our interviewees entered a realm in which women's concerns were raised in a more directly politicized way: several of the publications emanating from members of the organization have specifically articulated the needs for resources for women (for example Thomson and O'Sullivan, 1992). None of our respondents narrated their personal experiences from an explicitly feminist angle. In this way they were rather different from women involved as volunteers in organizations who were not themselves HIV-positive. In our study of volunteering at the Centre, we found that a relatively high proportion of women identified as lesbian or bisexual and saw HIV as a political issue connected both with their minority sexuality (and in support of gay men) and with women as women.

What this suggests is that the gendering of HIV for the individual cannot be divorced from that person's wider identification in social and community terms. And these identifications may change, related to a number of factors such as whether a woman's time and energies have to be devoted largely to child care or can be more widely spread. Since HIV is potentially so isolating and stigmatizing, identification with some form of support network becomes extremely important. Support and self-help groups, as we have seen, play a very important part in connection with a variety of chronic illnesses. The peculiar grouping of strongly negative cultural meanings attaching to AIDS makes the need for support, if anything, greater still. In conclusion, one can argue that the individual experience of HIV and AIDS can only be fully understood in wider and changing social contexts. It is the relationship between individuals and these contexts that is the key to understanding experience.

In sum, this chapter has illustrated how the experience of HIV/AIDS differs from experiences of living with other chronic illnesses, largely because of the stigmatization of AIDS through association with despised identities. The strong association between HIV/AIDS and gay men clearly influences their experiences of living with HIV/AIDS. The experiences of women in relation to AIDS are less marked in terms of identity, yet we have seen that, as with other illnesses, discrimination against women linked with their gender has material consequences for them. Inequalities based on such social divisions and gender, class and ethnicity will affect living with HIV/AIDS as it will living with any other debilitating illness. Conversely, many of the features of other chronic illnesses such as retrospectively giving meaning to symptoms on diagnosis, disassociation, passing and normalization can be seen in AIDS as well. In developing the general argument of this book, I propose that it is where AIDS interlocks with aspects of contemporary identities that it presents itself as a unique phenomenon. In other words, where aspects of people can be linked with aspects of AIDS as a late-modern social phenomenon and locus of fear, something different is created from the normal run of chronic illnesses. In Britain, therefore, it is gay men (and, to some extent, IDUs) who bear the greatest burden of the meanings of AIDS. These meanings are, however, not fixed, and in the concluding chapter I wish to review how the face of AIDS is changing in Britain in the late 1990s.

Notes

1. Our study was conducted in inner London, having among the highest prevalence rates for HIV in Britain. In low-prevalence areas HIV was generally less likely to be considered as a possible explanation for illness by GPs.
2. Recently (since 1996) decisions about testing have been influenced by the availability of new, relatively effective combination therapies, a subject I discuss in Chapter 6.
3. A progressive shift of funding from care to treatment in the late 1990s is reducing the level of such services available. See Chapter 6.
4. Breast cancer may also occur in men, but very rarely.
5. A tumour is said to have metastasized when cancerous cells have broken off and established new tumours elsewhere in the body.

6

Rethinking AIDS, Identity and Practice

This book has been an argument about AIDS as a social phenomenon expressive of contemporary identity anxieties. The trajectory of my analysis has concerned a specific historical moment and location: London in the early 1990s. I have considered individual and social experiences of AIDS in what might loosely be termed a symbolic interactionist perspective, illustrating a multiplicity of levels and meanings of AIDS in relation to identity expression. I have emphasized conscious, interactive, and intentional aspects of identity, a microsociology of identity in which identity is a prospective enterprise rather than a core residue of early childhood embroidered by adult experience. In concluding, I wish to tease out the implications of this analysis. To what extent does it raise theoretical, methodological and practical issues relevant beyond its historical frame? To answer this question I need to examine the late 1990s to set a context for this discussion.

At the end of the 1990s identities lie at the centre of a new politics, a politics in which the old divides of left and right and social class are obscured. The New Labour government, in its invocation of a 'Third Way', symbolizes Britain's contemporary, hard-to-classify political style. AIDS perhaps is fading from public consciousness: new treatments are available, the possibilities of effective vaccines seem nearer and it is less a subject of public fear and loathing. The continued relevance of AIDS to identity debates may be questionable, depending on the extent to which it is changing as a social phenomenon.

For reasons set out in the Introduction, the intersection of AIDS and identities has been examined largely via sexualized identities. For consistency I continue this perspective to examine the context of the end of the century. This chapter is structured therefore as an examination of how AIDS is changing, followed by a review of some recent analytical work on sexual identities and how these might be changing at century's end. Finally, with this context in place I will outline what in my analysis amounts to historical record, and what may be taken forward in research and in practical issues concerned with HIV/AIDS services and the needs of different groups.

AIDS at the end of the century

My analysis has concerned the experience of AIDS for individuals and localized groupings of individuals in London. The context in which AIDS is experienced is of course influenced by wider social, policy and medical agendas. In thinking about shifts in the meanings and significance of AIDS, I will consider recent notable changes in the medical and legal contexts of AIDS in the UK and how these may influence the experience of AIDS as a social phenomenon.

Virginia Berridge's *AIDS in the UK* (1996) provides a comprehensive analysis of the development of this 'macro' context in Britain between 1981 and 1994. Hers is an explicitly historical account. Commentaries concerning the same historical developments are also provided by Bennett and Ferlie (1994) and Garfield (1994), the former from an organizational and management theory perspective, and the latter in a more journalistic vein.

The early years until 1986, as Berridge and other scholars portray them, were marked by fear, ignorance, and bottom-up campaigning for a national response from voluntary groups, notably gay groups. The years 1986–7 saw the public health campaigning response of the then Conservative government, characterized by Berridge as being like mobilization in wartime (Berridge, 1996, Part Two). The 1990s might be described as a period of progressive normalization in a number of areas, though the process has been a complex one, not free of factions, rivalries and contests over the definition of AIDS as a problem and what should be done about it.

Personal experiences of AIDS have been influenced by this wider history, reflected in some of the narratives quoted in earlier chapters (for example, isolation and poor treatment by medical and nursing staff in the mid-1980s). By the mid-1990s the response to AIDS had become more diverse and dispersed than in the previous decade:

> The situation in 1994 was complex. The liberal consensus, the 'one-nation' ethos of the late 1980s was changing. But that had been a 'one-nation' stance founded on the defence of individual rights. The new consensus also emphasized the whole community, but in a way which subtly conflicted with the rights of the individual, as for example over testing and contact tracing. (Berridge, 1996, p. 278)

This quotation is significant in a number of respects. First, it encapsulates the historian's critical and scholarly approach to the evidence. Berridge's analysis brings to focus the range of forces that shaped Britain's experience of AIDS. So, whereas Mrs Thatcher is popularly construed (at least by what might loosely be termed the 'liberal left') as the basilisk who commanded Britain's most reactionary and philistine government this century (an image I find hard to dislodge, being a liberal lefty in my twenties in the 1980s), Berridge shows that the early coalition of interests around AIDS was not dominated by Thatcher's style. Indeed, a liberal consensus dominated in which medical professionals, among them notable gay men, worked in concert with gay AIDS activism and key civil servants. The reactionary aspect of Thatcherism had less impact than might be imagined, with the notable exception of her derailing of the planned national sex survey in the late 1980s (influenced by Kenneth Baker, David Mellor and Kenneth Clarke).[1] Examining the repoliticization of AIDS in the early 1990s, Berridge again paints a more nuanced picture than the 'degaying and regaying' argument put forward by gay campaigning groups such as GMFA, which I have described in Chapter 4. What she notes about this particular period is that pressures for regaying were accompanied by a broader-based change in perspective in which it was argued AIDS should be seen in a wider perspective of sexual health in the 1990s, and that HIV/AIDS services should therefore be offered via generic health and social services rather than as a specialism. The latter position, reflecting a complex of concerns for reducing costs, ensuring equity with other services, and de-stigmatizing AIDS, was not necessarily in conflict with a demand for more resources for gay men, but in practice the situation became a contradictory one in which marginalizing and mainstreaming tendencies were held in tension (*ibid.*, pp. 7–8).

Berridge's book is a valuable resource for examining the range of historical forces that have shaped Britain's experience of AIDS, and one that is carefully divorced from partisan expressions of interest. Her comment on the nature of a new consensus by the mid-1990s is useful in examining the situation at the end of the decade. The idea of a cross-community interest is in concert with the mainstreaming of AIDS services, but its significant difference from the early 1980s is in its valuing of community over individual in a way that echoes some aspects of Scandinavian public health approaches where the common interest is always placed above individual interest. Very recent developments in Britain support Berridge's thesis. In the judicial sense, individual responsibility to protect the common good is receiving greater emphasis, and the mainstreaming of services is being taken in new directions through the health and economic implications of the new combination therapies for AIDS.

The law and wilful transmission of HIV

In Cuba the state can quarantine people found to be HIV-positive. In Sweden, doctors must advise patients who are HIV-positive to practise safer sex, and if they refuse to do so or are discovered not to have done so, it is the doctor's legal responsibility to report the patient to the authorities, who may then detain him or her. Although in very different political contexts, both these national responses represent a valuing of community health over individual health to an extent that the end is seen to justify the means. Until recently, such measures were widely seen in Britain as draconian at least, fascist at worse. They were certainly opposed by most voluntary ASOs, and the liberal consensus which Berridge describes for the 1980s also found such measures distasteful and unacceptable.

In 1998 what might seem an extraordinary shift in this position has happened. On 11 February Home Affairs minister Alun Michael published draft legislation that would criminalize the deliberate transmission of disease with intent to cause serious harm. The law would apply to HIV, other sexually transmitted diseases and certain other infectious agents. This particular legal change is worth detailed attention, since the issue raised considerable controversy on its passage from a proposal of the Law Commission to legislation which has the support of a number of key ASOs in Britain, including the Terrence Higgins Trust.

A first obvious question is why did a call for such legislation arise in the first place? The Law Commission published its Consultation Paper No. 139 which raised the issue of criminalizing deliberate HIV transmission in late 1995, calling for responses from interested parties by June 1996 (later extended to December 1996). Until this time there had been no specific law in the UK concerning the transmission of HIV, but there had been cases where it was treated as a criminal offence under general laws, or as an aggravation of some other offence (such as rape or other assault). The impetus to bring about change came from a number of high-profile cases reported in the media in which someone claimed to have been deliberately infected with HIV by a sexual partner, through assault with a hypodermic syringe, or via invasive medical procedures. Several successful prosecutions had been brought in the USA, in one case after an HIV-positive man had spat at a police officer (the charge being attempted murder!; see Closen, Isaacman and Wojcik, 1993). In Britain the most publicized cases concerned Roy Cornes, a Birmingham man accused of deliberately infecting a number of female partners in the mid-1990s and a woman who, after living in London for several years, settled in rural County Cork and allegedly infected a number of local men. This second case is of particular interest because it richly illustrates the 'explosion of signification' which Paula Treichler (1988) associates with AIDS (as discussed in Chapter 3).

The circumstance of the revelation of this story was the confession of the woman to Father Kennedy, the priest in Dungarvan, that she was deliberately having unprotected sex with local men as 'revenge' for being infected with HIV by a man. Father Kennedy, viewing the matter as of grave seriousness to the local community, set aside the sanctity and confidence of the confessional and revealed the woman's behaviour, together with a description of her physical appearance, during his Sunday morning sermon.

The press treatment of this story, in September 1995, is full of images linking AIDS with sexuality, immorality and marginality in the ways discussed in Chapter 1. Even if we set aside tabloid responses, the so-called quality broadsheets are replete with dire prognostications stated in baroque, if not gothic, language. To take two examples, on 13 September the *Independent* ran a story in its *Life* section by Mary Braid and Ian MacKinnon with the headline 'Myth of the AIDS Avenger' subtitled 'A priest claims a woman has infected 80 men in an Irish village. Horror story or tall tale?' This might give the impression of a rational dispassionate investigation to follow, but even if this is the intention, the language used echoes the mystification of AIDS attacked by Susan Sontag, as described in Chapter 3. The opening paragraphs read:

> There have been terrifying reports of Aids [*sic*] Avengers before: homosexual men deliberately infecting partners with the HIV virus [*sic*], motivated by twisted revenge or blind fury at their own diagnosis. There were reports of mad American dentists deliberately injecting patients with their own infected blood in some horror-film parody. But yesterday an Irish priest, courtesy of the tabloid press, gave us the first female version of the Aids [*sic*] Avenging monster.
>
> According to Father Michael Kennedy, a promiscuous, tattooed, HIV-positive blonde has been marauding through Dungarvan, near Cork, like the Angel of Death, liberally spreading sexual favours among the village's young men and knowingly infecting up to 80 of them. The girl [*sic*], 25, who had recently arrived in the village from London, is reported to be 'demented' by her condition.

Maggie O'Kane's piece for the *Guardian* on 14 September occupies about 50 per cent of the front page, with the text under a large photograph of a pensive Father Kennedy beside the graveyard of his parish church. Her title is 'The Priest, the Angel of Death and the whispered distress of a small Irish town', byline 'Maggie O'Kane on the Aids [*sic*] torment of Dungarvan'. She describes the priest's revelation to his congregation on 10 September 1995 thus:

> At 10.30 last Sunday morning, Fr Kennedy stood under the buttercup yellow eaves of the parish church and, after he had preached his sermon on the importance of the celibate priest, told his town that he had something very serious to share with them.
>
> The church fell silent and still as a cat before the fatal pounce. Dungarvan had, he said, played host to an Angel of Death who

had sown her bitter Aids [*sic*] seed among their menfolk, infecting at least nine of them in six months. Afterwards, Fr Kennedy would say that the 25-year-old Londoner had come to Dungarvan for peace and anonymity but, unable to leave her anger behind, she had taken her lovers. They were young men from the towns of Youghal, Cork, Thurles and Dungarvan.

O'Kane went on to explain the likely incoherences in this version of events, as did Alan Murdoch in the *Independent* on 15 September. The probability of a woman transmitting HIV to so many men through unprotected sex was extremely low. And the South Eastern Health Board in Ireland threw doubt on the story since there had been no increased reporting of cases of HIV or AIDS in the region. This is aside from other problems common to such stories, most often that someone claiming to be infected by a particular source in fact had been exposed, or may have been exposed, to HIV elsewhere (most claims to infection by medical and dental practitioners have been discredited on these grounds).

The language used in the two articles quoted, though probably aimed at parody of tabloid coverage, reflects an inability or unwillingness to treat AIDS neutrally. The statements also encapsulate dominant popular images of AIDS. In the Dungarvan case it can even be argued that AIDS is used as a metaphor for rural Ireland, and, by implication, Britain in relation to Ireland. The woman alleged to be deliberately infecting men is variously identified as being English, and having an English accent (Maggie O'Kane) or as London-Irish (Murdoch). Her relative worldliness and association with the British metropolis is contrasted with the innocence of young rural Irish men. This patronizing image of Irish innocence is repeated in various registers: note the contrast between the disclosure in the sermon and the focus of the sermon on sexual continence (celibacy for the priest in relation to married heterosexuality for good Catholics). Then again, the imagery of good and evil, sin and sanctity, are all too crudely portrayed in phrases such as 'Angel of Death' and 'bitter AIDS seed'. The association between illness, sexuality, death and deviance is very clearly marked. The added ingredients of Catholicism and an implied relation between urban British fleshpots and rural Irish victimhood merely add a particular flavour. We are also told by O'Kane, irrelevantly, that Fr Kennedy is distantly related to a notable family of that name in the United States (third cousin to JFK) and that he recited the prayers for the dying at the bedside of Rose Fitzgerald Kennedy, matriarch. This may be bio-graphical detail, but is hardly neutral and further glamorizes and sensationalizes the story. O'Kane also describes Fr Kennedy as a 'fine born, handsome man' who, like the protagonist in the *Thorn Birds* (of which, we are told, the Father has a copy in his office) is bred to be the good Irish priest. Note that the priest in the televised version of *Thorn Birds* was played by Richard Chamberlain, who was also Dr Kildare in the popular television series. The intended associations are all too clear.

Stories about alleged deliberate transmission of HIV tend to gain attention when they are likely to attract readers, viewers and listeners; when they can create a sensation and invoke people's worst fears. In the lead-up to legislative change in 1998 two stories which went public attracted considerable media attention. In the summer of 1997 a scare erupted at an army barracks in Catterick, North Yorkshire. Several army personnel had had sex with local townswomen (sometimes described as 'prostitutes' in press coverage) who were reportedly HIV-positive. In the ensuing panic all servicemen based at the barracks were offered HIV antibody testing and counselling. None who tested was found to be positive (indeed one has subsequently become engaged to one of the accused women, and the story has largely been forgotten). As in the Dungarvan case, allegedly marginal women were demonized: promiscu-ity is a well known, even celebrated aspect of army life, yet the blame here was firmly placed on the women for potentially threatening the lives of 'healthy young men' serving their country. In the cases described so far, the subordinate treatment of women is clear, reflecting the discussion of AIDS and gender in Chapter 5.

The case that most directly influenced the Law Commission was that of a British woman, Jeanette Pink, who was infected with HIV by her Cypriot lover, Paul Georgiou. Georgiou was aware of his HIV status at the time, and was jailed by a Cyprus court for 15 months in August 1997. The evidence seemed fairly unequivocal in this case that infection could not have been caused by any other person at any other time. Pink, whose decline in health added to the poignancy of the case, argued that others like herself should be protected by law in future. A change in law could mean a deterrent to deliberate or reckless infection of others, and some chance to limit further infection in the case of a successful prosecution.

Pink put emphasis on these aspects of the law, rather than retributive justice. As a single, middle-aged woman who apparently had found sexual satisfaction and romance while on holiday, she was the subject of considerable public sympathy, tinged no doubt by echoes of the movie *Shirley Valentine*.[2]

The initial proposals in the Law Commission paper were that deliberate *and* reckless transmission of HIV should be criminal offences, carrying a maximum sentence of life imprisonment. The Law Commission recognized that HIV could be transmitted either maliciously or recklessly in circumstances in which physical assault was not involved, and that such cases under existing law could not be prosecuted. In the case of Jeanette Pink, reckless transmission could be invoked. Her partner knew he was HIV-positive, but did not disclose this information and she had unprotected sex with him believing him to be HIV-negative. In the Dungarvan case, ignoring the evidence contradicting the original story, it could be argued that the woman involved had deliberately and maliciously sought to infect men with HIV through having consensual sex with them. Under British law such a case could not be prosecuted at that time, with the added complication that in law a woman is not recognized as capable of raping a man, because she has no penis with which to penetrate (a point raised in arguments against the Law Commission proposals; see below).

The Law Commission, by reference to empirical evidence, pointed out what they saw as a gap in current law regarding the deliberate or reckless transmission of diseases likely to cause considerable harm. Since this gap existed in circumstances where consent had apparently been given (in the case of HIV, consenting sex or needle sharing) the focus of the legal case, as articulated explicitly in relation to HIV, had to be that intent or recklessness invalidated consent, in other words that the person giving consent had been misled (e.g. by a lie about HIV status) and therefore did not know that they were consenting to the possibility of being infected with HIV. This proposal was a significant modification of earlier notions of invalidation of consent. Previously, consent was only seen to be nullified if a fraud occurred that went to the nature of the act or the identities of persons involved. In the words of the Law Commission:

> We are, however, very concerned about one specific class of case ... We are referring here to the case where a person agrees to allow another to have sexual intercourse with him or her after that other person has untruthfully said that *he* has been tested for HIV

or other sexually transmitted diseases and that the findings were negative. It seems to us that this type of fraudulent misrepresentation is *morally different from* a fraudulent promise to pay for sexual services, and that it comes close to affecting the nature of the act itself in that it deals with matters that can have a physical consequence. We will be asking, therefore, whether a fraudulent misrepresentation that a person has had a test for HIV and/or other sexually transmitted diseases should form an exception to the general rule that fraud should nullify consent only where it goes to the nature of the act or the identity of the other person or persons involved in the act, and if so, in what terms this new class of misrepresentation should be formulated, and whether there are any other specific types of misrepresentation that also call for extraordinary treatment. (Law Commission, 1995, paragraph 6.19, p. 66, emphasis added)

A range of interested organizations responded to the Law Commission's proposals. These included the British Medical Association, Local Authorities and HIV/AIDS voluntary organizations. At the time, nearly all these bodies opposed, partially or completely, the new proposals. Their criticisms can be categorized as the following major types:

- A flawed understanding of the nature of sexual acts, in which a sex act is conceived as something done by one individual to another.
- A possible public demonization of persons living with HIV which in the long-term would discourage HIV antibody testing.
- Consequent on this demonization, that local and health authorities would be stymied in their statutory obligations to meet local HIV-related health and social needs.
- The proposals run counter to the public health tradition in Britain of education and voluntary testing/treatment of sexually transmitted diseases. They also conflict with the major governmental, medical, nursing and voluntary sector responses to HIV/AIDS developed since the mid-1980s.
- Cases of intentional and reckless transmission of HIV are in practice extremely rare.
- Proving beyond reasonable doubt that HIV transmission was deliberate is virtually impossible.

- Proving forensically that transmission could only have occurred from the defendant to the plaintiff is difficult.

I will consider each of these in turn, but first it is worth noting that cutting across these criticisms are two major themes:

(a) That the proposals are objectionable *in principle*.
(b) That the proposals will not result in any benefit. They have no *utility*.

Taking the example of demonization, the measures may be unacceptable in principle because they could lead to the further stigmatization of the HIV-positive and infringement of civil rights. On the other hand, they are of no benefit because they might discourage people from testing, thus endangering their own health and contributing to the *unintentional* spread of HIV. In this case principle and utility are compromised. Where the number of likely cases is considered, there could be a principled argument that deliberate infection of someone else with a potentially lethal virus should entail retribution by the law, but, given that only one such case has ever been proven beyond reasonable doubt throughout the world since the isolation of HIV, there seems hardly any point in doing it. Here it is utility alone that is compromised. Again, if we take proof of intent, both elements can be discerned. In the case of a private sexual act between two persons with no witnesses, the case amounts to one person's word against another's (albeit perhaps with supporting forensic evidence). The proposal has no utility if intent cannot be proven – the case would be thrown out of court. But this difficulty also raises an issue of principle: given the difficulty of proving intent, it would be extremely difficult to distinguish malicious from genuine prosecutions.

The law's conceptualization of sexual acts was taken to task by the BMA AIDS Foundation. Their argument was that this conceptualization was faulty and consequently biased the interpretation of intent and responsibility. In law a sexual act is assumed to be something done by someone to someone else, most usually by a man to a woman, involving penile penetration. The BMA indicated this was a very narrow view of sex and sexuality, and one premised in an active/passive dichotomy. They would prefer to see sex as an interaction of two persons, and therefore of two intentions, involving negotiations about what each partner wants to do. In the words of the cliché, it takes two to tango. In any sexual encounter that is consensual, it is sensible to see any outcomes as the product of two wills, for which both (or more) partners bear equal responsibility (BMA Foundation for AIDS, 1996, p. 4). This should apply to HIV exposure, among other things. Given almost universal public knowledge about the existence of HIV and how it can be transmitted, the BMA believed that anyone practising unprotected sex with a risk of exchanging body fluids must accept that they *may* be exposing themselves to risk of HIV transmission. The BMA also pointed out that different individuals have divergent ideas about what levels of risk they may be facing in any particular social situation, and what kinds and levels of risk they are prepared to expose themselves to. A sexual encounter is therefore a complex situation, which should never be reduced to a 'doer' and a 'done to'.

Further to this, the BMA argued that the potential harm engendered by exposure of HIV-positive status means that an HIV-positive person should not be legally obliged to disclose HIV status to sexual partners. In holding this position, the BMA wished to avoid scapegoating of the HIV-positive and call into question the category of 'reckless' transmission of HIV (*ibid.*, p. 9).

Voluntary sector HIV/AIDS organizations were particularly concerned at the negative impact the proposed legislation might have on HIV testing. With the availability of improved treatments (which I discuss below) the prevailing consensus among such organizations is that HIV antibody testing is now advisable for anyone who believes they may have been at risk of exposure to HIV. Current opinion is that HIV begins its deleterious work in the body long before symptoms become apparent, and that prognoses are improving with the new therapies, but that early treatment gives much better results than 'firefighting' at late stages of the illness. The fear for these organizations is that 'innocent' HIV-positive people might feel themselves open to malicious prosecution or discrimination by proxy (witch-hunts following sensational prosecutions). At the same time a disincentive for testing, running counter to personal and public health interests, might be created, since someone who was unaware of their HIV status logically could not be accused of deliberate transmission.

Both voluntary and statutory organizations involved in HIV prevention, care and treatment have raised concerns that their work might be impeded by the legislation. Fear of prosecution might drive people away from HIV-related services other than testing. This is a particular concern for health and local authorities, since they are required by statute to meet the health and social needs of their subject populations. Thus Hackney local authority in inner London, with a relatively high HIV-prevalence and populations deemed to be groups at risk, stated in its response to the Law Commission:

> If made law, we argue, such proposals would compromise the Council's role in provision of HIV care and prevention initiatives and services for those individuals, families and communities most disproportionately affected by HIV and AIDS and who already face substantial discrimination and prejudice. Furthermore, such proposals, if made law, we argue, would undoubtedly produce a legal barrier which would have a negative impact on our working in effective partnerships with those communities from our voluntary sector partners most affected and infected whom the Department of Health have described as 'originators of many of the innovatory services ... in prevention, treatment and care'.
> (London Borough of Hackney, 1996, para. 2.3, p. 2)

> Also there may be a change in how Council officers are perceived by those communities most affected by HIV and AIDS, away from a perception of being confidential towards a perception of reporting about clients' and service users' sexual behaviour and 'lifestyle'. This would reduce our ability to effectively provide services to those communities most affected and would problematise our targeting of HIV prevention initiatives to those individuals, families and communities at greatest risk, which we understand is not the intention of the Law Commission proposals.
> (*ibid.*, para. 4.5, p. 4)

A range of statutory and voluntary organizations pointed out that the legislation contradicted the general ethos of public health measures in Britain. They argued in particular that the system of education and voluntary testing in relation to STDs had been shown to work very well. This had its origins in the Royal Commission on the Venereal Diseases of 1917. A move towards involving the criminal law was fulfilling Berridge's prognosis of consensus moving from the protection of the individual to the protection of the public via individual sanctions.

> A key feature of the voluntary approach has been to encourage personal responsibility on the part of everyone, be they HIV negative, HIV positive or untested. The Law Commission's proposals represent a significant change of direction, in that they place an explicitly heavier burden of responsibility on individuals who are HIV positive, backed up by criminal sanctions. (BMA Foundation for AIDS, 1996, p. 1)

This point was argued contra the United States, where criminal legislation had led to violations of human rights and expensive litigation (as in the charge of attempted murder for spitting mentioned previously) and where a Cincinnati man with AIDS was beaten by four policemen and later charged with four counts of attempted murder for bleeding on his attackers. He was fitted with an electronic monitoring device on leaving hospital so police could track his whereabouts (Lurie, 1991).

All responses to the Law Commission emphasized the rarity of examples of deliberate transmission of HIV. Most alleged cases, as I have illustrated earlier, are not what they may seem at first and are frequently sensationalized. The vast majority of HIV-positive people are very concerned about the possibility of passing on the virus, as were all the interviewees in our research. On these grounds special treatment of HIV by criminal law may seem hardly worthwhile.

The final group of complaints, raised across the various organizations who responded to the proposals, focus on the fact that successful prosecutions are only a remote possibility, even where deliberate transmission has occurred. The latency period between infection and symptoms is such that retrospective identification of the occasion of infection is extremely difficult. The latency period between infection and production of antibodies (about three months) means that this difficulty exists even where someone gets an HIV antibody test immediately after an episode in which they think they may have been infected.

Proof that an action is intentional (as opposed to reckless) is, logically, virtually impossible. It would therefore be difficult to detect a malicious prosecution, and it is not unreasonable to think that a jury would tend to sympathize with the supposed 'victim'.

Viral genetic sequencing is becoming more commonly available, so transmission of a particular HIV strain from one person to another *is* now provable. But even this leaves problems over consent. The probability of successful viral transmission in any one act of sexual contact is small and unpredictable, as currently known to epidemiology. Neither the previously nor newly infected partner can reasonably predict that infection will occur on any particular occasion. This argument could be used in defence against the accusation of consent being invalidated. If probability enters the equation, consent can no longer be a zero-sum game.

The difficulties in bringing successful prosecutions led Angus Hamilton, a solicitor working on gay-related issues, to say that:

> The Government has changed the law in response to a very minor problem. The nature of HIV makes it very difficult to determine exactly when you were infected and by whom. Very few of these cases are going to get off the ground. (*Pink Paper*, 20 February 1998, p. 9)

In addition to these complaints, some of the respondents also discussed the meaning of 'serious injury' in relation to HIV transmission. These arguments are rather more abstract, and less relevant here since complainants agreed with the Law Commission that becoming infected with HIV was reasonably considered a serious injury.

All responses were otherwise generally critical of the proposals. The London Borough of Hackney argued they should be dropped altogether. The BMA AIDS Foundation argued that the criminal law should only apply in a set of very narrowly defined circumstances, namely:

- *either* the defendant has deliberately misled the plaintiff about his or her HIV status
- *or* the defendant knew that the plaintiff was positively mistaken (about the defendant's HIV status) in the sense of having expressed to the defendant a conscious belief which the defendant knew to be false
- *and* that the defendant knew or ought reasonably to have known that the plaintiff would not have given consent to sex had he or she been aware of the true facts. (BMA Foundation for AIDS, 1996, p. 10)

These proposals rule out reckless transmission, but accept that deliberate transmission should be seen as a crime.

In February 1998 a modified version of the original proposal from the Law Commission was incorporated in a green paper and draft bill to replace the Offences Against the Person Act, for debate in Parliament in the autumn session. The matter of HIV transmission was only a minor element in a wider attempt to replace an outdated and ineffective area of criminal justice. In addition, the legislation would only apply to deliberate (not reckless) transmission and would apply also to other infectious agents that may cause serious illness.

It was widely expected that the new legislation would be passed, and a precedent had already been set by the success of similar legislation in the Republic of Ireland. The public announcement of the proposed legislation was endorsed by all the major HIV/AIDS voluntary organizations, most notably the Terrence Higgins Trust, whose director, Nick Partridge, appeared on national television to say that the THT supported the move, and that he was satisfied the law would not and could not be used to criminalize otherwise innocent HIV-positive people. The National AIDS Trust took a similar position. The only ASO that has totally condemned the legislative proposals has been the George House Trust in Manchester.

Given the initial negative reactions to the Law Commission proposal described earlier, this might at first sight appear to be a U-turn. The reasons for the change centre on an acceptance that the legislation will more narrowly, rather than more broadly, define grounds for prosecution, and that there is an argument to be made in terms of the public good for prosecuting deliberate infection of others. A defining example supporting this position is the case of Ian Dagger. This man was accused of trying to infect someone with a syringe of HIV-contaminated blood. Transmission of the virus did not result but if it had, under prior legislation it would have only been possible to prosecute him for causing a needle prick, not transmitting HIV. The far greater (potential) harm would have slipped the net of the law (Julian Meldrum, National AIDS Trust, personal communication). A public call for punishment of deliberate HIV transmission is not in itself unreasonable. Indeed the BMA had pointed out in its original submission that the concern for change in the law was less about public health (the likely numbers involved being so small) than about a moral objection to people freely and deliberately infecting others with a potentially lethal virus, in which case the law should apply to other infectious agents (BMA Foundation for AIDS, 1996, p. 5). This leaves open the question of whether the very fact of legislation might deter people from testing for HIV antibodies, in which case harm may result along the lines suggested by Hackney Council in its submission. On this matter, the major voluntary organizations tend to take the view that very few people would be put off testing if they are satisfied that the law will apply only to provable deliberate transmission (Julian Meldrum, National AIDS Trust, personal communication).

Whether or not the new legislation will have any effects on people living with HIV remains to be seen. It may well be, as Angus Hamilton suggests, a storm in a tea cup. Qualitative research of the sort described in this book might provide insight into the effects of the legislation for the person living with HIV, whatever these may be. The point remains that whether or not we see prosecutions for HIV transmission and fear of prosecution among the HIV-positive, the legislation is part of a move towards a moral consensus that legislation should protect the common good more than the rights of the individual, and that this is part of a wider shift in political ethos in Britain in the late 1990s.

New treatments and the end of AIDS?

> there has been little consideration of the ways in which the new virology will affect HIV prevention policies and practice. This paper argues that it will inevitably result in unprecedented upheavals. Even if the effectiveness of today's therapies is still insufficient to bring to fruition the more optimistic aims, such as totally halting disease progression or even curing infected people, the fact that these possibilities are now openly discussed in medical circles itself has implications for HIV prevention work. In the UK treatment issues have usually been ignored or overlooked by the AIDS voluntary sector. Now more than ever it is essential that HIV prevention workers understand the significance of recent medical advances and prepare for the impact on their work. (King, 1997, p. 13)

Edward King addressed his concerns here to HIV prevention, but his themes are relevant to treatment and care as well. Current evidence indicates that the new antiviral therapies, their costs and therapeutic value, will considerably alter the terrain of AIDS, and what living with AIDS means.

Chief among the new anti-HIV drugs, available for clinical treatment since 1996, have been the protease inhibitors. The first three of these released for prescribed use were saquinavir, ritonavir and indinavir (trade names Invirase, Norvir and Crixivan, respectively). These protease inhibitors were shown in clinical trials to have far greater inhibitory effects on HIV than the earlier nucleoside analogue drugs such as AZT, 3TC, ddI and ddC. It was also found, however, that because of the propensity of HIV to mutate, each drug used alone soon became ineffective as resistant HIV strains emerged. But if two or more drugs were administered together as a 'cocktail' the overall effect was both greater and much more sustained. 'Combination therapy' was shown to reduce viral loads in the blood dramatically, and to result in remarkable improvements in health in a significant number of cases (*ibid.*, pp. 16–18). The evidence from virology suggested that the combination therapies would be most effective for someone newly infected with HIV, when the virus has had little time to mutate drug-resistant strains, and the immune system is relatively intact. Indeed the possibility was raised of destroying the virus altogether after several years of therapy, in other words that HIV becomes curable. It was also argued that someone at a later stage of infection might considerably benefit from combination therapy in the sense of a much improved prognosis.

To date, the evidence about the therapies is equivocal. Some people who made remarkable recoveries at first have subsequently become ill or died. Others cannot tolerate the drugs. They clearly are not a panacea. They are, though, the most significant therapeutic advance since the beginning of the AIDS epidemic in 1981. They have considerable future ramifications.

Some of their implications relate to HIV prevention. As Edward King describes, if HIV becomes curable, then post-exposure prophylaxis may be possible, in which case concepts of risk and safer sex will change (*ibid.*, pp. 26–7). Most significantly, in relation to prevention, HIV/AIDS voluntary organizations have moved towards broad recommendation of HIV testing for anyone who thinks they may have been at risk of exposure. If the therapies are effective, and most effective when started soon after infection, the benefits of finding out you are HIV-positive may outweigh the disadvantages, since HIV may no longer be seen as a possible or likely death sentence and, if curable, should no longer be a cause of stigma or discrimination.

In the context of this book my interest is more in the implications of the combination therapies for the meaning of HIV and AIDS in the lives of people who are already knowingly HIV-positive. Two themes can be discussed. First, there are shifts in policy surrounding provision of treatment and care services, which will have a material impact on the lives of the HIV-positive. Second, there are the self-perceptions of HIV-positive people – how they believe their lives will change because of the effects of the new therapies (effects being clinical, social and political).

Policy on the provision of treatment and care is being affected by two interrelated factors. First, the National Health Service is experiencing a resource crisis. And the new combination therapies are currently very expensive. The Inner London Health Authorities estimated that these drugs might cost them as much as £50 million in 1998/99 (ILHHCG, 1997, p. 4). Combination therapy provision will have to be at the cost of cuts in other services. Second, there is a general pressure, continuing what Virginia Berridge identified in the mid-1990s, towards the mainstreaming of HIV services, reducing unit costs and (so the National Health Service hopes) lessening the stigmatization of HIV. The advent of the new drugs has itself played into mainstreaming: the need for inpatient care should be reduced and it is hoped, in line with the move towards community care, that in future more HIV-positive people will receive most of their treatment from their GP rather than hospitals or GUM services (Winn, 1997).

The details of changes in services in the immediate future are made clear by the Inner London HIV Health Commissioners' Group (ILHHCG) in their Framework for the Purchasing of HIV and GUM Services for 1998/99. This group co-ordinates HIV/AIDS health service purchasing across inner London in concert with local authorities where community care policy requires joint working of health and social services. Their position tends to be precedent-setting for the UK as a whole, since inner London contains the highest concentration of HIV cases in the nation.

In the context of the mainstreaming of HIV services and a general need for rationalization and efficiency, the framework document specified that services would only be purchased in future if they followed the over-arching objectives of:

- the diagnosis of HIV infection and other sexually transmitted diseases
- the treatment of conditions which result from HIV infection and sexually transmitted diseases
- the maintenance of health of adults and children diagnosed with HIV
- enabling adults and children with HIV-related illness to be supported in the community, as appropriate. (ILHHCG, 1997, p. 4)

As well as these overarching objectives, there is a general move towards residence-based funding, that is that health authorities will fund services only for their own residents rather than on an open-access basis, and that service providers, in order to secure funding, must increasingly demonstrate that the effectiveness of their services is shown by evidence.

In practice these objectives would mean that inpatient, outpatient and day care/treatment services, GUM services and NHS Community Health Services would continue to be funded, though with some structural changes and deletions. Major cuts, though, were anticipated for community care services jointly funded by the NHS and local authorities. Broadly defined, these are the kinds of services provided by voluntary sector organizations such as the Centre in my study, described in earlier chapters. Advice services such as housing advice, legal advice and welfare rights advice would be reduced by funding fewer providers and using more restrictive definitions of the services and who would constitute a legitimately qualified practitioner. Counselling services would also be reduced by funding fewer providers and at lower unit costs. Drop-in services which, as I have argued earlier, formed a crucial component of self-help at the Centre, will face considerable cuts, unless they are a route of access to other services. Their open access basis will also be eroded by the move towards residence-based funding of services. Complementary therapies will not be funded at all by ILHHCG, though they state that individual authorities may still purchase such services as part of local provision (*ibid.*, p. 2). The reason given for this cut is that such services have never been purchased consistently across inner London, so are not appropriately part of ILHHCG's remit. The rather thin evidence base for the effectiveness of complementary therapies might also be a factor. Again, as I have discussed earlier, complementary therapies were perceived by users of the Centre as a very important therapeutic component of their experience of the Centre. Such therapies were so valued that the Centre has recently raised funds from charitable sources to cover the anticipated cuts.

The reorganization of HIV/AIDS services and the financial impact of the new combination therapies will inevitably have a negative effect on social care organizations such as the Centre. On 6 March 1998 the *Pink Paper* announced that the London Lighthouse, the highest-profile HIV and AIDS care centre in Britain, was about to enter crisis talks with the Department of Health after a reduction of health authority funding of £1.7 million compared with the previous year. Already the number of beds and nurses had been cut. A week later it was announced that the organization was to sell its prestigious West London building.[3] It is generally agreed that these cuts are driven by the costs of the new therapies, yet in the absence of evidence that therapies work for everyone or indefinitely for anyone, the HIV voluntary sector forecasts dire consequences for people living with HIV.

As I have argued in earlier chapters, the Centre was valued by its users as much for providing a safe environment in which to explore and share the meanings of living with HIV as for the direct benefits of individual services available there. This, I would argue, reflects the profound social meanings of HIV and AIDS beyond illness. Currently such services are facing swingeing cuts when HIV and AIDS have not yet come to be seen by the general public in neutral terms, as just another health need among many. The attention given to the criminalization of deliberate HIV infection makes this clear. If such services are cut wholesale then a void will exist for many HIV-positive people, and the normalization of AIDS to the point where it is generally seen as another manageable chronic illness of no particular note is still some way off.

Personal reactions to the new therapies and changes in service provision by people living with HIV have not yet been extensively researched. Much of the commentary is anecdotal and relayed via voluntary sector organizations (see Anderson and Weatherburn, 1998, p. 4), though a limited amount of detailed research is beginning to be published. A number of organizations, including London Lighthouse, have begun organizing support and training sessions for HIV-positive people anticipating a return to work. In the past, an HIV diagnosis plus debilitating illness would, as I illustrated in Chapter 3, sometimes lead to a withdrawal from work and an expectation that the rest of one's life would be lived on benefits. The new therapies are changing this. Now, improvements in health of such a degree have happened that someone may physically be able to return to work, and of course the state would expect him or her to do so if possible. Various outcomes might result for the individual. A return to work might enable a considerable enhancement of self-esteem. On the other hand, for someone who has been ill for years, a forced return to work may be a very daunting prospect. Being out of the labour market for many years could make it difficult to find work at all, or only work at a much lower status level than previously enjoyed (compare Anderson and Weatherburn, 1998, p. 36). Furthermore, for someone living on full benefits, to carry on living at the same standard might mean finding a job with a salary in excess of £20,000 per year: this is unlikely after prolonged absence from work.

Preliminary qualitative research in which HIV-positive people were interviewed about their expectations of the future has been conducted by Will Anderson and Peter Weatherburn for SIGMA Research. In this six-month pilot study they conducted in-depth semi-structured interviews with 25 gay men and 15 African men and women who had been using combination therapy for at least four months. These interviews considered clinical and social impacts of the therapies, and reveal a diversity of individual and group experience against a background of uncertainty connected with the novelty of the therapies.

> The changes in health (for better or worse) which therapy brings will mean radically different things to different people, however similar their clinical circumstances. Everyone's life brings together a unique past, a complex present and a set of hopes and expectations for the future. It is only in this context that the impact of therapy can be understood. (*ibid.*, p. 6)

In spite of the diversity, Anderson and Weatherburn were able to identify significant patterns. The gay men were generally better informed about HIV, more likely to know someone else with HIV and able to access support via their social networks and HIV/AIDS services. The Africans typically experienced more isolation and discrimination in their own communities, and were diagnosed as HIV-positive relatively late. In these respects the differences between gay men and Africans echo my earlier findings in the evaluation of the Centre.

The patterned responses to the new therapies were categorized by Anderson and Weatherburn as follows:

- Quiet self-preservation
- Investing in a new future
- Bewildered by hope
- Enjoying early retirement
- New hope is too much risk
- Keeping momentum despite everything

The *quiet self-preservers* saw the therapies as offering better and longer life prospects, but not a miracle cure. They recognized that years of illness had taken a toll on their resources, and that the regimen for the new therapies demanded time and discipline, as well as the therapies them-selves having debilitating side effects such as nausea. Those *investing in a new future* were experiencing positive results of treatment and were very optimistic about future life prospects. Their will for life was radically transformed into a sense of regained self (as I have described in Chapter 3). They recognized the uncertainties but were prepared to take risks. People *bewildered by hope* also saw new possibilities, but found them frightening when their lives had been dominated by the prospect of illness and early death. In their case new prospects meant anomie (a lack of recognized norms) rather than hope. The familiar life landscape was transformed to another country.

Enjoying early retirement and *new hope is too much risk* resembled quiet self-preservation and bewilderment by hope, respectively, but with significant biographical differences. Like the quiet self-preservers, those enjoying early retirement had optimism for the future, but with the expectation of a life built around leisure activities rather than any attempt to return to a working life. These people were generally older, or had been HIV-positive for a considerable time. Those who felt that the *new hope was too much risk* also perceived improved future prospects, but at the expense of losing a certain security founded on enhanced benefits and social and health support from HIV services. They did not, however, experience the same degree of apprehension as those bewildered by hope.

Some interviewees had always maintained a positive attitude to living with HIV and had accommodated it as far as possible with minimum disruption to their lives. For these people the new therapies represented a continuation and enhancement of this approach, which amounted to *keeping momentum despite everything.*

Overall, this research is optimistic about the early outcomes of novel treatments, but is careful to indicate the wider and sometimes contradictory effects, effects very different for different individuals and groups. The authors in particular pay attention to the implications for working life:

> Undoubtedly the dominant ethos was in favour of work, but only a few people saw having work as of unqualified benefit – for most, work had its attractions and its disincentives. For those who were not employed, returning to work was rarely perceived to be a critical goal, thanks both to the many obstacles to getting work and to the existence of alternatives. There were also those who had decided that their paid working lives were over and were happy to enjoy (early) retirement. (*ibid.*, p. 35)

Such individual responses were conditioned and constrained by wider social and structural factors. Thus, Africans with unclear immigration status may not be entitled to benefits and are therefore forced to work if possible. A relatively older gay man in a good pension scheme might have early retirement as an easy option. Always the individual and the social are interlaced.

These experiences echo some of the responses to life with HIV that I have discussed in Chapter 3, yet they suggest possibilities that couldn't exist at the time of the evaluation of the Centre. Both optimism and fear enter new registers. More research of the kind conducted by Anderson and Weatherburn will be needed if we are to understand the social impact of combination therapy as it is progressively improved and normalized within the experience of HIV.

The new antiviral treatments will likely have a much greater impact on the lives of the HIV-positive than the legislation around deliberate HIV transmission. They change the whole environment in which life with HIV is to be lived (assuming their continued success). Those becoming newly infected with HIV may not find it the life-changing scenario I have painted in earlier chapters. Those who have lived with HIV for many years may find the future landscapes of their lives changed beyond recognition. This may be positive, the finitude of life may expand for them once more, but it also may mean trying to regain something thought forever lost. It might leave behind a generation of people whose personal and social losses have been tremendous, and who may feel their pain is forgotten by those who come later and for whom HIV holds much less dread.

What I have been describing are general changes in the political, social and clinical context in which HIV exists, which may significantly alter the experience of HIV for anyone who is positive. The main interest in this book has been in the relation of HIV and AIDS to identities, but more particularly I have focused on sexual identity and HIV/AIDS, and most of my evidence has concerned gay men and AIDS. I also began by situating my arguments about AIDS in wider debates about the nature of modernity and the contemporary significance of sexual identities, especially in the West. To continue the theme of how the relationship between AIDS and identities may be changing as we approach the millennium, I consider now some recent debates about the future of gay identities.

The end of the modern homosexual?

Lesbians and gay men have been the recipients of considerable media attention in the late 1990s. In the general election of 1997 two newly elected Labour MPs, Stephen Twigg and Ben Bradshaw, had stood as openly gay candidates. Then later in the year a junior minister, Angela Eagle, came out as lesbian. In 1994 a vote in Parliament on the lowering of the age of consent for gay men from 21 to 16 was narrowly defeated, resulting in a compromise reduction to 18. Equalization with heterosexual consent at 16 was again given a free vote on 22 June 1998, and this time, with a large Labour majority in government, the amendment to the Crime and Disorder Bill was passed with a majority of 207 votes.[4] The amendment was later voted down in the House of Lords, but it was guaranteed to pass into law eventually since the government, in the light of rulings by the European Court of Human Rights, decided to adopt equalization of the age of consent as government policy through a single-clause bill in the autumn 1998 session of Parliament.

Various other campaigns articulated around notions of equality and citizenship show signs of bearing fruit. The lesbian and gay equality campaigning group Stonewall continue to argue for the lifting of a Ministry of Defence ban on homosexual personnel in the armed forces, for equal partnership rights in the workplace for homosexual as well as heterosexual couples, and for the broader recognition of same-sex relationships, the latter to include parenting and inheritance rights. Some campaigners have gone further, to ask for the institution of marriage to be extended to same-sex couples (see Sullivan, 1995).

Legislation in Britain seems to be moving in the direction of slowly accepting lesbians and gay men as full citizens, although yet another forum for gay equality has recently been formed (The Equality Alliance). At the same time, attitude surveys suggest that the condemnation of homosexuality is gradually lessening among the general population, though still prominent in Britain. Younger people, particularly the 16–24 age group, are slightly more tolerant than the rest of the population (Johnson *et al.*, 1994, p. 241), which may be indicative of a trend beyond a general tendency of the young to be more liberal than their elders. Such changes have to be viewed critically. The most positive changes are in line with legislative changes; the idea that all citizens should be treated equally and have the right to conduct their lives as they please, so long as they don't harm anyone else. This is not the same thing as saying that dislike of homosexuality is disappearing. In the *Sexual Attitudes and Lifestyles* study published in 1994, taking a random sample of 20,000 people throughout Britain, 70.2 per cent of men and 57.9 per cent of women said that they believed sex between two men to be always or mostly wrong (*ibid.*). Furthermore, homosexuality is still seen as different and marginal where questions of family are concerned: most people still disapprove of lesbian or gay male couples being able to foster or adopt children.

Homosexuality, nevertheless, has become a subject widely discussed and reported on. It is frequently discussed in the media, and the volume of programming aimed at a primarily lesbian and gay audience continues to increase, for example the magazine series *Gaytime TV* on Channel Four. There is an optimism among lesbians and gay men as never before that life will get better.

There are arguments, as I said earlier, that AIDS is heading towards some form of normalization within society, not least if it becomes more effectively treatable. A parallel question is also being asked of whether homosexuality isn't also becoming normalized, and what consequences may flow from this. A paradox is suggested. If same-sex sexual orientation comes to be seen as normal, then what happens to lesbian and gay identities, since these are surely forged out of a sense of difference?

This theme is at the centre of much current debate in lesbian and gay studies within the social sciences and cultural studies over the future trajectory of lesbian and gay identities. Among social constructionists, most argue that being lesbian or gay is not simply an expression of an inherent sexual tendency but a culturally and historically specific reaction to the ways Western society characteristically conceptualizes sexuality and sexual identity. Just as historical and cultural conditions produced lesbians and gay men, so might they make them redundant. Some social scientists argue precisely that this is happening. Lesbian and gay identities simply won't be necessary in future. Paradoxically, essentialists can adopt the same position. If they can show that homosexuality is simply part of the natural variation in genetically controlled human sexuality, then there is no reason from within a scientific rationalist position to treat homosexuals any differently from heterosexuals. The orientation in itself need not be seen as a fundamental source of difference; a special identity category, or rather categories of lesbian and gay, are no longer needed. Yet there are others who would argue that there is historical evidence of condemnation of homosexuality in most human societies through most of history. Homophobia and compulsory heterosexuality are not going to disappear overnight. This group tend to see historical change as being much slower, and that lesbian and gay identities are concrete and likely to remain necessary for some considerable time to come. These arguments are all, of course, political as much as they are academic, since they have importance for the way that people live their lives and the rights they effectively have in relation to the rest of society.

The debate about the future of lesbian and gay identities hinges on how they are seen to link with the conditions of modernity. Chapter 1 discussed how sexual identities are argued as being expressive of modern conditions. In concluding my examination of identity I want to address some of the work which proposes that sexual identities will change as a result of shifts in modernity.

Gay identities and the homosexual form of existence

A key text on the relations between modernity and sexuality, updated and translated into English in 1997, is Henning Bech's seminal *When Men Meet* (published originally in 1987, in Danish). This work argues that what Bech terms 'the homosexual form of existence' is made possible by social conditions in late modernity, indeed that homosexuality represents a concentration of the forces of modernity, is an archetype of modernity. Others, such as Tim Edwards, have proposed that we are experiencing a fragmentation of identities coeval with the postmodern condition (Edwards, 1994). Whether one prefers postmodernism or late modernity as explanatory trope, the trend in analysis for the future of gay identities is similar.

Bech begins by suggesting that although social constructionism has added much to the study of sexuality, it has several flaws. In using the concept of identity it tends to overplay the separation between the gay man and other men. The gendered category of masculinity, recognized in much anthropological study of sexuality as a key component of sex–gender systems, gets partially or totally ignored in favour of considering relations between identities and erotic object choice. Furthermore, identity-focused social constructionism does not consider the relations between non-homosexual men and homosexuality. To avoid this pitfall, Bech proposes two related concepts:

(a) the homosexual form of existence
(b) proclaimed (gay) identities

He is not interested in the origins of same-sex desires, nor in who does and does not have them, and takes these as given. Sociologically, he posits that modernity makes possible the homosexual form of existence, which in turn has led to the possibility of proclaimed gay identities. But the latter does not necessarily follow from the former. There may be people who participate in the homosexual form of existence, but who do not perceive themselves as having a gay identity. The distinction is useful in relation to HIV prevention and the category labelled MSM, which belongs in (a) but not (b). It is also useful in relation to my usage of identity throughout this book. Largely I have used it as equivalent to proclaimed gay identity. But what precisely does Bech mean by the distinction?

There have been throughout history and most human cultures men who have desired sexual contact with other men. Before the advent of modernity, Bech argues, such contact either had to be fleeting, or was structured around differences in male status, such as the Athenian citizen (*erastes*) and his boy lover (*eromenos*). Only in modern societies have conditions arisen where men of equal status can freely and frequently associate sexually. It is the modern city that provides the space in which this can happen: a relatively anonymous existence among a large and highly mobile population (Bech, 1997, p. 112). Bech uses the urban railway station, typically a cruising ground, to symbolize the city as a sexualized space. People come out into the city as a space in which to be homosexual. They need to do this because homosexuality is reviled, and in a peculiarly modern way.

Modernity reproduces itself through the patriarchal nuclear family. Homosexuality does not fit here and must establish itself away from community of origin and family ties. In this sense, homosexuality is different. Yet it crystallizes wider aspects of modernity. As I related in Chapter 1, modernity is widely conceptualized as characterized by choice and insecurity. The homosexual merely experiences a lack of traditional role more acutely:

> The homosexual, then, is close to the uneasiness that clings to modern existence in general: the impossibility of becoming one with what one is, the compulsion constantly to play a part. He is a born existentialist and a practising role-theoretician. (*ibid.*, p. 97)

Once in the city, and having accepted being homosexual, the homosexual can pursue the homosexual form of existence. This is available both as sexual contact and as more nuanced social association.

> Being together with other homosexuals allows one to mirror oneself and find self-affirmation. It allows one to share and inter- pret one's experiences. It allows one to learn in detail what it means to be homosexual: how to act, what to think, thus lending substance to one's proclaimed identity, as well as assimilating certain techniques that may help bridge the gap between this identity and one's actual experiences and conduct. (*ibid.*, p. 116)

Here is the key link between homosexual form of existence and gay identity. Gay identity only exists as a conscious project forged with others who share the homosexual form of existence. In this book I have tried to show how proclaimed identities have coalesced around AIDS. As I have not been closely interested in sexual practice and sexualized spaces (at least not in this book) the concept of the homosexual form of existence has played a much smaller role. It is important, however, in thinking about the future of gay identities.

The homosexual form of existence is a modern phenomenon. It was produced by modernity. For Bech modern life first affected homosexuals, but he sees these effects as extending elsewhere in modern societies. For example, homosexuals have had the opportunity to be freely sexual, and to contract relationships which are egalitarian, of mutual benefit, and only need last as long as they are beneficial (compare Giddens, 1992). This is in contrast with traditional heterosexual marriage in which many argue that women were always treated as the property of men. With increasing divorce rates and increased unwillingness to enter marriage in the first place, heterosexual relationships are tending to resemble homosexual ones. In Bech's terms, a homosexualization of society is happening.

At the same time the master discourses that pronounce on sexuality, particularly psychiatry, have decided that homosexuality is not pathological, and cannot be cured. Given modern society's general regard for medicine, this should lead to greater acceptance of homosexuality. In both social and medical terms, then, what was regarded as peculiar to homosexuality is disappearing. Bech predicts that the modern homosexual may soon disappear as a species and that same-sex preference may come to be seen as a matter of taste rather than something of great import (Bech, 1997, p. 209). With the disappearance of the homosexual form of existence, gay identities will no longer be necessary, and they will gradually evaporate as sources of individual and group identification.[5]

Bech's conclusion is controversial. In response to criticism, he has acknowledged that modernity is less homogeneous than he paints it. The normalization of homosexuality may be much more advanced in his home country, Denmark, and elsewhere in Scandinavia than in, say, the United States or Britain. In a discussion of these ideas at a conference on the cross-cultural study of sexuality (University of Amsterdam, July 1997) American participants argued that identification around an implicit ethnicity was salient in the USA with a history of civil rights politics, and that Queer Politics continued successfully in a society where sexual difference was still strongly proscribed. Compulsory heterosexuality and homophobia have not gone away. British participants argued that the situation in Britain is probably closer to the United States than Denmark. Acceptance of registered partnerships or same-sex marriage is much further off here than in Scandinavia (Denmark has already accepted registered same-sex partnerships).

Whoever is right, and whatever the differences between countries, we cannot assume that being a gay man will continue to have either the content or the force it currently possesses in relation to identity. Where we are interested in AIDS we must see that while the meanings of AIDS are changing, the meanings of being gay may also change, independently. A future study of the kind I have reported in this book may find a very different relationship between sexual identity and AIDS, and possibly a less distinct and powerful one.

To interrogate the mire of shifting and overlapping identities and communities, we might follow the suggestions of Anthony Cohen and Donna Haraway. Cohen, in thinking about community from the perceptions of members and outsiders invites us to focus on the symbolic boundary. To those outside, a community may appear fairly homogeneous: to those inside, it will be marked by difference (Cohen, 1985). Any examination of community needs to take these multiple perspectives into account and look at how insider and outsider dynamics interact, particularly if those on one side of the boundary have resources which those the other side don't. We should also consider how in pursuit of political goals those inside a community may deliberately and consciously downplay difference (Deverell and Prout, 1995, p. 208). This is one way of looking at the way community claims of gay activists have worked, as discussed in Chapter 4.

The development of individual identities might best be thought of in terms of affinities, rather than overarching identities. Criticizing the reifying instincts of 1980s feminism, particularly the assumption that being a woman implies a shared identity with other women, Donna Haraway (1990) suggests that we dispense with the concept of identity in any totalizing or essential sense. Instead we can look at how aspects of identity lead to the forming of specific affinities and allegiances in historical and cultural context. We can look then at how forms of identity and community are chosen, negotiated and achieved. In terms of a political project this opens up a space for forging unities while not erasing difference.

Rather than this being an outright rejection of the concept 'identity', I see it as a useful modification that can help in explaining the connections between particular empirical outcomes and a theoretical perspective capable of encapsulating them. Affinities developed within and across the symbolic boundaries of community are what we might look for in future explorations of identity.

Examining identities and AIDS: prospects

In closing I wish to offer some observations on the particular versus general relevance of the research presented in this book. The particular relations between proclaimed sexual identity and AIDS described are historically specific. In this chapter I have outlined significant changes in the meanings of AIDS and possible changes in gay identities, which reinforce the conviction that my analysis is historically specific. On the other hand, I can argue that its theoretical stance and methodology are valid and should continue to be used in future studies of identity and of AIDS and other chronic illnesses.

I argued in Chapter 2 that identities (proclaimed identities in Bech's terms) have important performative aspects. To capture these, a research methodology ideally should include some component of participant observation, as well as other qualitative research instruments such as semi-structured interviews. Although I did not use them myself, focus groups are also relevant, since they allow social processes of attitude and knowledge formation to be made visible through the interaction of group members. It is argued that they are an ideal way of observing the cultural construction of experience (Wilkinson, 1998), though they tend to obscure marginal voices pushed aside by dominant group members.

I have also argued that the investigation of chronic illness should include individual and group components. Most of the sociological literature to date focuses methodologically on the individual, even if it asks questions about impacts on primary relationships, social networks, and so on. In my analysis of the Centre I have suggested more partici- patory research techniques to look at how the chronically ill experience their illness socially. Such methods are relevant to looking at other illnesses. In this book I have tried to concentrate on exploring how AIDS is or is not different from other chronic illnesses. If AIDS (I hope) disappears or at least shrinks because it becomes treatable or at least manageable, the kind of analysis I have conducted can still be repeated for conditions that remain intractable, especially where they link with identities (for example, gender-specific illnesses).

In the context of provision of services to particular groups in society affected disproportionately by serious illnesses, the research methods remain relevant. The rhetoric of care in the community asserts that the service user must have a voice in which services are provided, how and to whom (a special issue of *Community Care: Research Matters* in summer 1998 reports on user involvement in a variety of social care contexts). Direct representation by users in health authorities, local authorities and NHS Community Care Trusts is one way to achieve this. Recording and presenting user voices in a way that does not constrain them is also possible through evaluative research of the kind I have described. I have presented individual voices of group members, and group members articulating a voice as a group. This kind of research can present the authentic concerns of groups of service users without first framing research from a social problem perspective. This differentiates it from research directly commissioned by or for service providers, who generally set out from a perceived problem for which they want a solution, for example 'why are not as many black people using our services as we would like or as we would expect from the epidemiology for this illness in this location?' These are valid questions, but as they assume a problem to begin with, they may miss out on some wider dynamic of the situation.

Last, I have suggested that identity is in part about making claims. Health authorities and social services tend to assume that people have needs; and they then have a statutory obligation to meet those needs. Things are not that simple. What is a need and who has it are open to ideological interpretation and manipulation, as we saw in Chapter 4. A quite sophisticated knowledge of how people operate is needed to disentangle the needs that institutions are legitimately meant to meet from those that service users can lay claim to. Needs develop in context, they are not something lying out there waiting to be discovered. Needs assessments are the bread-and-butter of current service provision and spending decisions. They may not always be worth the paper they are written on.

Notes

1. This survey was originally proposed by the Health Education Authority and Social and Community Planning Research. Potential Department of Health funding was withdrawn by the government, but the study was eventually funded by the Wellcome Trust and published as *Sexual Attitudes and Lifestyles* (Johnson *et al.*, 1994).
2. *Shirley Valentine* was a popular film made in 1989, written by Willy Russell, produced and directed by Lewis Gilbert, and starring Pauline Collins as Shirley and Tom Conti as her Greek lover Costas.
3. Later in 1998 the organization raised sufficient funds to keep the building, but had to close the residential unit.
4. For a thorough analysis of the gay age of consent debate in Britain from a social constructionist perspective, see Waites, 1996, 1998.
5. Bech's whole analysis of homosexuality depends on its relationship with a concept of masculinity. We are not told, therefore, what the future may hold in store for lesbians.

References

Adam, B. (1992) 'The state, public policy and AIDS discourse', in J. Miller (ed.), *Fluid Exchanges*. Toronto: University of Toronto Press.

Adam, B. and Sears, A. (1996) *Experiencing HIV: Personal, Family and Work Relationships*. New York: Columbia University Press.

Alcorn, K. (1992) 'Communities of the night', *Capital Gay* (London), 18 September, p. 14.

Altman, D. (1986) *AIDS and the New Puritanism*. London: Pluto Press.

Altman, D. (1994) *Power and Community: Organizational and Cultural Responses to AIDS*. London: Taylor and Francis.

Anderson, W. and Weatherburn, P. (1998) 'The impact of combination therapies on the lives of people with HIV'. Research Report. London: Sigma Research.

Annetts, J., Eisenstadt, K. and Gatter, P. (1996) *Gay and Bisexual Men's HIV Prevention Service Review and Social Mapping Project. Final Report*. London: Lambeth, Southwark and Lewisham Health Authority.

Bebbington, A., Feldman, R., Gatter, P. and Warren, P. (1992) *Evaluation of the Landmark: Final Report*. Discussion Paper 901/2. Canterbury: University of Kent, Personal Social Services Research Unit.

Bebbington, A. and Gatter, P. (1994) 'Volunteers in an HIV social care organization', *AIDS Care*, 6(5), 571–85.

Bech, H. (1997) *When Men Meet: Homosexuality and Modernity*. Oxford: Polity Press.

Beck, U. (1992) *Risk Society: Towards a New Modernity*. London: Sage.

Bell, D. and Valentine, G. (eds) (1995) *Mapping Desire: Geographies of Sexualities*. London: Routledge.

Bennett, C. and Ferlie, E. (1994) *Managing Crisis and Change in Health Care. The Organizational Response to HIV/AIDS*. Buckingham: Open University Press.

Berridge, V. (1996) *AIDS in the UK: The Making of Policy, 1981–1994*. Oxford: Oxford University Press.

Blasius, M. (1994) *Gay and Lesbian Politics: Sexuality and the Emergence of a New Ethic*. Philadelphia: Temple University Press.

BMA Foundation for AIDS (1996), *Response to Law Commission Consultation on Consent in the Criminal Law*. London: British Medical Association.

Born, G. (1994) 'Anthropology, psychoanalysis, and the subject in culture.' Unpublished seminar paper. London: University College, Medical Anthropology Series.

Boswell, J. (1980) *Christianity, Social Tolerance, and Homosexuality: Gay People in Western Europe from the Beginning of the Christian Era to the Fourteenth Century*. Chicago: University of Chicago Press.

Brandes, S. (1981) 'Like wounded stags: male sexual ideology in an Andalusian town', in S. Ortner and H. Whitehead (eds), *Sexual Meanings*. Cambridge: Cambridge University Press.

Bury, M. (1982) 'Chronic illness as biographical disruption', *Sociology of Health and Illness*, 4(2), 167–82.

Butler, J. (1989) *Gender Trouble: Feminism and the Subversion of Identity*. New York: Routledge.

Butler, J. (1993) *Bodies That Matter: The Discursive Limits of 'Sex'*. New York: Routledge.

Cain, R. (1994) 'Managing impressions of an AIDS service organization: into the mainstream or out of the closet?' *Qualitative Sociology*, 17(1), 43–61.

Cant, B. (ed.) (1997) *Invented Moralities? Lesbians and Gays Talk about Migration*. London: Cassell.

Carpenter, E. (1894) *Sex-Love and Its Place in a Free Society*. Pamphlet. Manchester.

Carroll, L. (1888) *Through the Looking Glass*. London: Macmillan.

Charmaz, K. (1983) 'Loss of self: a fundamental form of suffering in the chronically ill', *Sociology of Health and Illness*, 5, 168–95.

Closen, M., Isaacman, S. and Wojcik, M. (1993) 'Criminalization of HIV transmission in the USA'. Paper PO D27 4188. Chicago: The John Marshall Law School.

Cohen, A. (1985) *The Symbolic Construction of Community*. London: Routledge.

Cohen, A. (1994) *Self Consciousness: An Alternative Anthropology of Identity*. London: Routledge.

Community Care: Research Matters (1998) User Focused Research. Special issue, August. Sutton: Reed Business Information.

Coward, R. (1989) *The Whole Truth: The Myth of Alternative Health*. London: Macmillan.

Crimp, D. (ed.) (1988) *AIDS: Cultural Analysis, Cultural Activism*. Cambridge: MIT Press.

Cunningham, D. (1977) 'Stigma and social isolation: self-perceived problems of a group of multiple sclerosis sufferers'. Report no. 27. Health Services Research Unit, University of Kent, Canterbury.

Darwin, C. (1859) *The Origin of the Species by Means of Natural Selection; or, The Preservation of Favoured Races in the Struggle for Life*. London: Murray.

Davis, F. (1963) *Passage through Crisis: Polio Victims and Their Families*. Indianapolis: Bobbs Merrill.

Davis, M., Klemmer, U. and Dowsett, G. (1991) *Bisexually Active Men and Beats: Theoretical and Educational Implications*. The Bisexually Active Men's Outreach Project. AIDS Council of New South Wales and Macquarie University AIDS Research Unit.

Davies, P. (1992) 'The role of disclosure in coming out among gay men', in K. Plummer (ed.), *Modern Homosexualities: Fragments of Lesbian and Gay Experience.* London: Routledge.

Dawkins, R. (1976) *The Selfish Gene.* Oxford: Oxford University Press.

Deverell, K. (1992) 'Leicester Black MESMAC: an evaluation of outreach work in saunas'. MESMAC Evaluation Working Paper no. 4. London: Health Education Authority.

Deverell, K. and Prout, A. (1995) 'Sexuality, identity and community – reflections on the MESMAC Project', in P. Aggleton, P. Davies and G. Hart (eds), *AIDS: Safety, Sexuality and Risk.* London: Taylor and Francis.

Douglas, M. (1966) *Purity and Danger.* Harmondsworth: Penguin.

Douglas, M. (1992) *Risk and Blame: Essays in Cultural Theory.* London: Routledge.

Douglas, M. and Wildavsky, A. (1982) *Risk and Culture.* Berkeley: University of California Press.

Edwards, T. (1994) *Erotics and Politics: Gay Male Sexuality, Masculinity and Feminism.* London: Routledge.

Ellen, R. (ed.) (1984) *Ethnographic Research: A Guide to General Conduct.* London: Academic Press.

Epstein, S. (1987) 'Gay politics, ethnic identity: the limits of social constructionism', *Socialist Review,* **93/94**, 9–54.

Epstein, S. (1996) *Impure Science: AIDS, Activism and the Politics of Knowledge.* Berkeley: University of California Press.

Evans-Pritchard, E. E. (1937) *Witchcraft, Oracles and Magic among the Azande.* London: Oxford University Press.

Fallowfield, L. with Clark, L. (1991) *Breast Cancer.* London: Routledge.

Feldman, R., Garside, R. and Gatter, P. (1996) *Research in AIDS Care: An Annotated Bibliography of Social Research in HIV and AIDS Care in the United Kingdom.* London: National AIDS Manual Publications.

Fitzpatrick, R. (1984) *The Experience of Illness.* London: Routledge.

Foucault, M. (1978) *The History of Sexuality. Volume 1: An Introduction.* Harmondsworth: Penguin.

Gamson, J. (1989) 'Silence, death and the invisible enemy: AIDS activism and social movement "newness" ', *Social Problems,* **36**, 351–65. Also in M. Burawoy (ed.), *Ethnography Unbound: Power and Resistance in the Modern Metropolis.* Berkeley: University of California Press (1991).

Gamson, J. (1996) 'Must identity movements self-destruct?: A queer dilemma', in S. Seidman (ed.), *Queer Theory/Sociology.* Oxford: Blackwell.

Garfield, S. (1994) *The End of Innocence: Britain in the Time of AIDS.* London: Faber and Faber.

Gatter, P. (1995) 'Anthropology, HIV and contingent identities', *Social Science and Medicine,* **41**(11), 1523–33.

Gatter, P. (1998) 'Policing boundaries: linking the theory and experience of psychotherapy in HIV/AIDS research', in R. Barbour and G. Huby (eds), *Meddling with Mythology: AIDS and the Social Construction of Knowledge.* London: Routledge.

Geddes, P. and Thompson, A. (1890) *The Evolution of Sex.* New York: Scriber and Welford.

Giddens, A. (1979) *Central Problems in Social Theory: Action, Structure and Contradiction in Social Analysis.* London: Macmillan.

Giddens, A. (1991) *Modernity and Self-Identity: Self and Society in the Late Modern Age.* Oxford: Polity Press.

Giddens, A. (1992) *The Transformation of Intimacy: Sexuality, Love and Eroticism in Modern Societies*. Oxford: Polity Press.

Goffman, E. (1963) *Stigma: Notes on the Management of Spoiled Identity*. Englewood Cliffs, NJ: Prentice-Hall. Also Pelican edition, Harmondsworth: Penguin Books, 1968.

Gorna, R. (1996) *Vamps, Virgins and Victims: How Can Women Fight AIDS*. London: Cassell.

Gupta, S. and Boffin, T. (eds) (1990) *Ecstatic Antibodies: Resisting the AIDS Mythology*. London: Rivers Oram Press.

Habermas, J. (1979) *Communication and the Evolution of Society*. Boston: Beacon Press.

Halperin, D. (1990) *One Hundred Years of Homosexuality, and Other Essays on Greek Love*. London: Routledge.

Halperin, D. (1997) 'Forgetting Foucault: acts, identities, and the history of sexuality'. Keynote conference address, 'Beyond Boundaries: sexualities across culture', 29 July 1997, University of Amsterdam, Netherlands.

Hammersley, M. (1992) *What's Wrong with Ethnography?* London: Routledge.

Haraway, D. (1990) 'A manifesto for cyborgs: science, technology, and socialist feminism in the 1980s', in L. Nicholson (ed.), *Feminism/Postmodernism*. London: Routledge.

Hardy, R. (1990) 'Risky business: confronting unsafe sex', *Village Voice* (New York), 26 June, pp. 35–8.

Heaphy, B. (1996) 'Medicalisation and identity formation: identity and strategy in the context of AIDS and HIV', in J. Weeks and J. Holland (eds), *Sexual Cultures: Communities, Values and Intimacy*. London: Macmillan.

Heaphy, B. (1998) 'Reinventing the self: identity, agency and AIDS/HIV'. PhD thesis, University of the West of England.

Herdt, G. (1983) *Ritualized Homosexuality in Melanesia*. Berkeley: University of California Press.

Herdt, G. (ed.) (1992) *Gay Culture in America: Essays from the Field*. Boston: Beacon Press.

Herdt, G. and Stoller, R. (1990) *Intimate Communications: Erotics and the Study of Culture*. London: Routledge.

ILHHCG (1997) 'Framework for the purchasing of HIV and GUM services for 1998/99: final draft'. London: Inner London HIV Health Commissioners' Group.

Johnson, A., Wellings, K., Wadsworth, J. and Field, J. (1994) *Sexual Attitudes and Lifestyles*. Oxford: Blackwell Scientific Publications.

Kayal, P. (1993) *Bearing Witness: Gay Men's Health Crisis and the Politics of AIDS*. Boulder, CO: Westview Press.

Kelley, P., Pebody, R. and Scott, P. (1996) *How Far Will You Go?: A Survey of London Gay Men's Migration and Mobility*. London: Gay Men Fighting AIDS.

Keogh, P., Beardsell, S., Hickson, F., Reid, S. and Stephens, M. (1995) 'The support and resource needs of gay men with HIV/AIDS, their partners and their carers. A report by Sigma Research to the Terrence Higgins Trust.' Portsmouth: Sigma Research, School of Health Studies, University of Portsmouth.

King, E. (1993) *Safety in Numbers*. London: Cassell.

King, E. (1997) 'HIV prevention and the new virology', in J. Oppenheimer and H. Reckitt (eds), *Acting on AIDS*. London: Serpent's Tail.

King, E., Rooney, M. and Scott, P. (1992) *HIV Prevention for Gay Men: A Survey of Initiatives in the UK*. London: North West Thames Regional Health Authority.

Kippax, S., Connell, R., Dowsett, G. and Crawford, J. (1993) *Sustaining Safe Sex: Gay Communities Respond to AIDS*. London: Falmer Press.

Knopp, L. (1995) 'Sexuality and urban space: a framework for analysis', in D. Bell and G. Valentine (eds), *Mapping Desire*. London: Routledge.

Kobasa, S. (1991) 'AIDS volunteering: links to the past and future prospects', in D. Nelkin, D. Willis and S. Parris (eds), *A Disease of Society: Cultural and Institutional Responses to AIDS*. Cambridge: Cambridge University Press.

Kramer, L. (1990) *Reports from the Holocaust*. Harmondsworth: Penguin.

Kubler-Ross, E. (1970) *On Death and Dying*. London: Tavistock Publications.

Law Commission (1995) *Consent in the Criminal Law*. Paper no. 139. London: HMSO.

Laws, S. (1990) *Issues of Blood: The Politics of Menstruation*. London: Macmillan.

Levine, M. (1979) 'Gay ghetto', in M. Levine (ed.), *Gay Men: The Sociology of Male Homosexuality*. New York: Harper and Row.

London Borough of Hackney (1996) 'Response to the Law Commission's Consultation Paper no. 139 "Consent in the Criminal Law".' London: Borough of Hackney.

Lurie, R. (1991) 'PWA charged with murder attempt for bleeding', *The Advocate*, 19 November.

Lynn, P. and Davis Smith, J. (1992) *The 1991 National Survey of Voluntary Activity in the UK*. Voluntary Action Research, Second Series, Paper no. 1. Berkhamsted: The Volunteer Centre.

Mac an Ghaill, M. (1996) 'Irish masculinities and sexualities in England', in L. Adkins and V. Merchant (eds), *Sexualizing the Social: Power and the Organization of Sexuality*. London: Macmillan.

McCormack, C. (1982) *Ethnography of Fertility and Birth*. London: Academic Press.

Mars-Jones, A. (1996) Film review in the *Independent* (London), 25 April.

Mercer, K. (1995) 'Imagine all the people: constructing community culturally', in National Touring Exhibitions, *Imagined Communities* exhibition catalogue. Manchester: Cornerhouse Publications.

Miles, A. (1979) 'Some psycho-social consequences of multiple sclerosis: problems of social interaction and group identity', *British Journal of Medical Psychology*, 52, 321–31.

Moore, H. (1994) *A Passion for Difference*. Oxford: Polity Press.

Moore, O. (1996) PWA Column, *Guardian Weekend* (London), 21 September.

Myslik, W. (1996) 'Renegotiating the social/sexual identities of place', in N. Duncan (ed.), *Body Space*. London: Routledge.

NAM (1994a) *Local Government, AIDS and Gay Men. Results of a Survey into the HIV and AIDS Services of Local Government in England and Wales, with a Particular Emphasis on Work with Gay Men and Bisexual Men*. London: NAM Publications.

NAM (1994b) *Health Purchasing, HIV Prevention and Gay Men. Results of a Survey into the Purchasing of HIV Prevention Work for Gay Men and Bisexual Men by Health Authorities in England*. London: NAM Publications.

National Audit Office (1991) *HIV and AIDS Related Health Services*. Report by the Comptroller and Auditor General. London: HMSO.

Ortner, S. and Whitehead, H. (eds) (1981) *Sexual Meanings: The Cultural Construction of Gender and Sexuality*. Cambridge: Cambridge University Press.

Patton, C. (1990) *Inventing AIDS*. London: Routledge.

Patton, C. (1994) *Last Served? Gendering the HIV Pandemic*. London: Taylor and Francis.

Peek, P. (ed.) (1991) *African Divination Systems: Ways of Knowing*. Bloomington: Indiana University Press.

Pelto, P. and Pelto, G. (1978) *Anthropological Research: The Structure of Enquiry*. Second edition. Cambridge: Cambridge University Press.

Plummer, K. (1995) *Telling Sexual Stories: Power, Change and Social Worlds*. London: Routledge.

Pollak, M., Paicheler, G. and Pierret, J. (1992) *AIDS: A Problem for Sociological Research*. London: Sage.

Prout, A. and Deverell, K. (1995) *Working with Diversity: Evaluating the MESMAC Project*. London: Health Education Authority.

Rajchman, J. (1991) *Truth and Eros: Foucault, Lacan and the Question of Ethics*. London: Routledge.

Robinson, I. (1988) *Multiple Sclerosis*. London: Routledge.

The Royal Society (1992) *Risk: Analysis, Perception, Management*. London: The Royal Society.

Ryan, L. (1995) ' "Going public" and "watching sick people" – the clinic setting as a factor in the experiences of gay men participating in AIDS clinical trials', *AIDS Care*, 7(1), 147–58.

Scambler, A. and Scambler, G. (1993) *Menstrual Disorders*. London: Routledge.

Scambler, G. (1989) *Epilepsy*. London: Routledge.

Schlesinger, P. (1987) 'On national identity: some conceptions and misconceptions criticized', *Social Science Information*, 26(2), 219–64.

Schramm-Evans, Z. (1990) 'Responses to AIDS: 1986–87', in P. Aggleton, P. Davies and G. Hart (eds), *AIDS: Individual, Cultural and Policy Dimensions*. London: Falmer Press.

Seidman, S. (ed.) (1996) *Queer Theory/Sociology*. Oxford: Blackwell.

Sharma, U. (1992) *Complementary Medicine Today: Practitioners and Patients*. London: Routledge.

Shuttle, P. and Redgrove, P. (1980) *The Wise Wound*. Harmondsworth: Penguin.

Sigma Research (1996) *Behaviourally Bisexual Men in the UK: Identifying Needs for HIV Prevention*. London: Health Education Authority.

Sobo, E. (1995) 'Finance, romance, social support and condom use among impoverished inner-city women', *Human Organization*, 54(2), 115–28.

Sobo, E., Zimet, G., Zimmerman, T., Jackson, J., Mortimer, J., Yanda, C. and Labeznik, R. (1995) 'Sexual behaviour, drug use and AIDS knowledge among midwestern runaways', *Youth and Society*, 26(4), 400–62.

Sontag, S. (1978) *Illness as Metaphor*. New York: Farrar, Straus and Giroux.

Sontag, S. (1989) *AIDS and Its Metaphors*. New York: Farrar, Straus and Giroux.

Sontag, S. (1991) *Illness as Metaphor* and *AIDS and Its Metaphors*. Harmondsworth: Penguin.

Stromberg, P. (1986) *Symbols of Community: The Cultural System of a Swedish Church*. Tucson: University of Arizona Press.

Sullivan, A. (1995) *Virtually Normal: An Argument about Homosexuality*. London: Picador.

Sutton, W. and Munson, T. (1976) 'Definitions of Communities: 1954–1973'. Paper presented at the American Sociological Association meetings, New York.

Tan, M. (1995) 'From *Bakla* to gay: shifting gender identities and sexual behaviours in the Philippines', in R. Parker and J. Gagnon (eds), *Conceiving Sexuality: Approaches to Sex Research in a Postmodern World*. London: Routledge.

Thomson, K. and O'Sullivan, S. (eds) (1992) *Positively Women: Living with AIDS*. London: Sheba Feminist Press.

Toufexis, A. (1995) 'New evidence of a "gay gene" ', *Time*, **146**(20), 13 November.

Treichler, P. (1988) 'AIDS, homophobia, and biomedical discourse: an epidemic of signification', in D. Crimp (ed.), *AIDS*. Cambridge, MA: MIT Press.

Vance, C. (1989) 'Social construction theory: problems in the history of sexuality', in D. Altman *et al.*, *Homosexuality, Which Homosexuality?* London: Gay Men's Press.

van Den Hoek, J., Van Griensven, G. and Coutinho, R. (1990) 'Increase in unsafe homosexual behaviour', *The Lancet*, **336**, 179–80.

Verres, R. (1986) *Krebs und Angst. Subjektive Theorien uber Ursachen, Verhutung, Fruherkennung, Behandlung und die psychosozialen Folgen von Krebserkrankungen*. Berlin, Heidelberg: Springer-Verlag.

Vincke, J., Mak, R., Bolton, R. and Jurica, P. (1993) 'Factors affecting AIDS-related sexual behaviour change among Flemish gay men', *Human Organization*, **52**(3), 260–68.

Waites, M. (1996) 'Lesbian and gay theory, sexuality and citizenship', *Contemporary Politics*, **2**(3), 139–49.

Waites, M. (1998) 'The age of consent and sexual citizenship in the UK: a history', in J. Seymour and P. Bagguley (eds), *Relating Intimacies: Power and Resistance*. Essays from the 1997 BSA Conference. London: Macmillan.

Watney, S. (1987) *Policing Desire: Pornography, AIDS and the Media*. London: Methuen.

Watney, S. (1993) 'Emergent sexual identities and HIV/AIDS', in P. Aggleton, P. Davies and G. Hart (eds), *AIDS: Facing the Second Decade*. London: Falmer Press.

Watney, S. (1994) *Practices of Freedom: Selected Writings on AIDS*. London: Rivers Oram Press.

Weeks, J. (1981) *Sex, Politics and Society: The Regulation of Sexuality since 1800*. London: Routledge.

Weeks, J. (1985) *Sexuality and Its Discontents*. London: Routledge.

Weeks, J. (1995) *Invented Moralities: Sexual Values in an Age of Uncertainty*. New York: Columbia University Press.

Weeks, J. (1996) 'The idea of a sexual community', *Soundings*, **2**, 71–84.

Weeks, J., Aggleton, P., McKevitt, C., Parkinson, K., and Taylor-Laybourn, A. (1996) 'Community responses to HIV and AIDS: the "de-gaying" and "re-gaying" of AIDS', in J. Weeks and J. Holland (eds), *Sexual Cultures: Communities, Values and Intimacy*. London: Macmillan.

Weitz, R. (1991) *Life with AIDS*. London and New Brunswick: Rutgers University Press.

West, P. (1986) 'The social meaning of epilepsy: stigma as a potential explanation for psychopathology in children', in S. Whitman and B. Hermann (eds), *Psychopathology in Epilepsy: Social Dimensions*. Oxford: Oxford University Press.

Wilkinson, S. (1998) 'Focus groups in feminist research: power, interaction, and the construction of meaning', *Women's Studies International Forum*, **21**(1), 111–25.

Winn, S. (1997) 'The role of the primary health care team in the care of people with HIV and AIDS', *Health and Social Care in the Community*, 5(6), 408–17.

Wrubel, J. and Folkman, S. (1997) 'What informal caregivers actually do: the caregiving skills of partners of men with AIDS', *AIDS Care*, 9(6), 691–706.

Index